Multiple Pregnancy - New Insights

Edited by Hassan S. Abduljabbar

Published in London, United Kingdom

Multiple Pregnancy - New Insights
http://dx.doi.org/10.5772/intechopen.101014
Edited by Hassan S. Abduljabbar

Contributors
Rafiea Jeddy, Mandefro Yilma Asfaw, Yakov Y. Yakovlev, Tshililo Mashamba, Jennifer Ayton, Emily Hansen, R. Kishore Kumar, B.R. Usha, Ramya Santhanam, Anandharama Subramani Padmanabhan, Navya Nanjundegowda, Hassan S. Abduljabbar

First published in London, United Kingdom, 2023 by IntechOpen
IntechOpen is the global imprint of INTECHOPEN LIMITED, registered in England and Wales, registration number: 11086078, 5 Princes Gate Court, London, SW7 2QJ, United Kingdom

British Library Cataloguing-in-Publication Data
A catalogue record for this book is available from the British Library

Additional hard and PDF copies can be obtained from orders@intechopen.com

Multiple Pregnancy - New Insights
Edited by Hassan S. Abduljabbar
p. cm.
Print ISBN 978-1-80356-197-4
Online ISBN 978-1-80356-198-1
eBook (PDF) ISBN 978-1-80356-199-8

Meet the editor

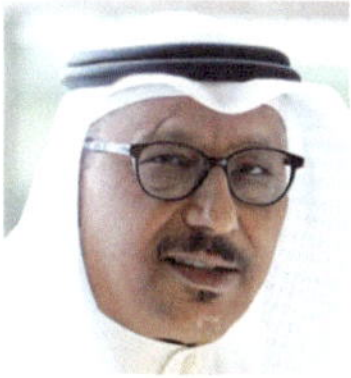

Professor Hassan S. Abduljabbar, MD, FRCSC, is president of the Federation of Arab Gynecology Obstetrics Societies. He obtained an MD from King Abdulaziz University College of Medicine and Allied Health Sciences, Jeddah, Saudi Arabia, in 1980. He became a fellow of the Royal College of Physicians and Surgeons of Canada in 1986 after four years of training at the University of Western Ontario, Canada. In 1988, he became board certified by the American Board of Obstetrics and Gynecology (ABOG). Dr. Abduljabbar is a referee for many international scientific medical journals. He is also an examiner for master's and postdoctoral degrees as well as the Saudi and Arab board exams. He has published more than seventy-five articles and edited six books.

Contents

Preface IX

Section 1
Introduction 1

Chapter 1 3
Introductory Chapter: About Multiple Pregnancies
by Hassan S. Abduljabbar

Chapter 2 11
Multiple Pregnancy: Boon or Bane – An Indian Perspective
by R. Kishore Kumar and B.R. Usha

Chapter 3 21
Types of Multiple Pregnancy
by Tshililo Mashamba

Chapter 4 31
Multiple Gestation
by Mandefro Yilma Asfaw

Section 2
Rare Diagnosis of Multiple Pregnancy 45

Chapter 5 47
Selective Intrauterine Growth Restriction in Monochorionic Twins
by Ramya Santhanam, Anandharama Subramani Padmanabhan and Navya Nanjundegowda

Chapter 6 61
Recent Updates in the Management of Monochorionic Twin Pregnancy
by Rafiea Jeddy

Section 3
Breastfeeding **93**

Chapter 7 **95**
Perceived Insufficient Milk Supply (PIMS) in Lactating Mothers
by Yakov Y. Yakovlev

Chapter 8 **103**
Breastfeeding Multiples
by Jennifer Ayton and Emily Hansen

Section 4
Complication **117**

Chapter 9 **119**
Complications of Multiple Pregnancy: Conception to Delivery
by Tshililo Mashamba

Preface

This book discusses multiple pregnancies and their incidence and risk factors.

Twins are the commonest type of multiple pregnancy. When twins develop from one zygote fertilized by one sperm and the zygote splits and forms two embryos, the twins are considered monozygotic or identical. When twins develop from two zygotes fertilized by two sperm, the twins are considered dizygotic or fraternal. One in 250 natural pregnancies will result by chance in twins.

Diagnosis of multiple pregnancies is done via medical history and physical examination. Quantitative beta-human chorionic gonadotropin (hCG) levels in twin pregnancies may be relatively high. An early ultrasound, around 6 to 10 weeks, can confirm the pregnancy and check for issues.

Patients with multiple pregnancies need more folic acid, calories, protein, and other nutrients. These patients should be referred to see a maternal-fetal medicine specialist.

The delivery method for a multiple pregnancy depends on many factors, including the babies' health, positions, and gestational age.

This book is organized into four sections. The first section is an introduction to multiple pregnancies, the second section describes the rare diagnosis of multiple pregnancies, the third section discusses breastfeeding, and the fourth and final section examines complications of multiple pregnancies and their management.

Hassan S. Abduljabbar
Professor,
Dr. Erfan and Bagedo General Hospital,
Obstetrics and Gynecology Department,
Jeddah Fertility Center,
Jeddah, Saudi Arabia

Section 1

Introduction

Chapter 1

Introductory Chapter: About Multiple Pregnancies

Hassan S. Abduljabbar

1. Introduction

Twins are the commonest type of multiple pregnancies. It means that two offspring created by the same pregnancy can be identical and become (monozygotic). Twins usually develop from one zygote, which splits and forms two embryos, non-identical or (dizygotic), meaning that each twin sets from separate oocytes, fertilized by different sperm [1]. One in 250 natural pregnancies will result by chance in twins [2].

2. Types of twins

The first type is when two separate oocytes are fertilized by two different sperm. This is non-identical or (dizygotic twins), but the result of if one oocyte fertilized, this is identical twins (monozygotic). Rare type is conjoined twins. There are rare (unique) twins, mirror twins, conjoined twins (physically connected.), parasitic twins, semi-identical twins, and female and male identical twins [3].

3. The risk factors

Genetics, diet, previous pregnancies, and use of fertility drugs are risk factors for multiple pregnancies and raise the chances of having twins. Age is another essential factor, especially ages over 35 have a greater chance of multiple pregnancies. High parity and race are risk factors [4]. Igbo-Ora, southwestern Nigeria, Twin Capital of the World, has a large number of twin pregnancies. In Igbo-Ora, research has suggested that this is most likely related to the women's eating habits in the area [5, 6]. Research has found no direct relationship between dietary intake and multiple pregnancies but has proven that a widely consumed tuber (yams) could be responsible [6, 7].

4. Multiple pregnancies are increasing

There has been about a 10-fold rise in twinning rates over the past two decades [8]. Around 30–50% of all twin pregnancies result from infertility treatments. The incidence of twins increased in the last four decades in developed countries. As women delayed childbearing and the age of the first pregnancy became late became an important factor, and wild use of medication for induction of ovulation and IVF increased the probability of multiple births [9].

5. Vanishing twin syndrome

About 10–15% of singleton births start as twins, and often, one is lost in the early pregnancy; this is called vanishing twin syndrome. In 1945, vanishing twin syndrome was first recognized [10, 11].

6. Cryptophasia

According to what is (published in the Journal Institute of General Linguistics), there are bizarre phenomena that twins can speak a unique language only they can understand. But it disappears with time as the twins grow and learn other languages [12].

7. Time of delivery

The percentage of twins that can make it to 37 weeks' gestation is 49%, and 6% are preterm [13]. Care is required during the antenatal period twin pregnancy is more susceptible to anemia; thus, they need extra care for their health and different prenatal vitamins. Women pregnant with twins should take the same prenatal vitamins for any pregnancy, but recommending extra folic acid and iron. The additional folic acid and excess iron will help ward off iron-deficiency anemia, which is more common when pregnant with multiple pregnancies [14].

The meaning of twin, A, and B The twin developing closest to the cervix is called Baby A, and the other is called baby B [15].

8. ART and Multiple pregnancies

Multiple pregnancies are now more common as a result of fertility treatments [16]. In vitro fertilization (IVF) might cause multiple pregnancies due to more than one embryo transfer [17]. Induction of ovulation non-ART fertility treatments stimulates the development of multiple oocytes, which cannot be controlled, and may lead to multiple pregnancies [18].

We know that some infertility patients prefer to have twins. Still, as a fact, all multiple pregnancies have higher risks for both infant and mother [19]. It has been shown that in the last four decades, multiple pregnancies steadily increased, and twins nearly doubled [20]. The increasing trend of multiple pregnancies coincides with the introduction of fertility treatment [21]. After considering maternal age, more than one-third of twins and more than three-quarters of triplets and higher-order multiples resulted from conception assisted by fertility treatments [22]. Improving the practice of ART results in a decrease in multiple pregnancies due to fewer embryos being transferred during ART [23].

The maximum number of embryo transfers should not be more than four in women above the age of 39 years. In those older women with high-quality embryos, no more than three embryos should be transferred. If four embryos are transferred, the data suggest that the transfer of four or more embryos has a positive effect: increasing the pregnancy rates without significantly impacting the multiple pregnancy rates. This effect is only seen in women aged <45. Transferring three embryos may increase the chance of multiple pregnancies without increasing the overall pregnancy rate. The maximum number of embryo transfers should not be more than three embryos [24].

Fertility treatments can cause twins to have a higher risk of congenital disabilities than singletons; it questions the notion that fertility treatments contribute to those abnormalities [25]. The implantation of two fertilized oocytes leads to twins, and requesting to transfer more than one embryo may increase the chance of multiple pregnancies [26].

9. There are risks associated with IVF twins

9.1 Preeclampsia

It is one of the complications of multiple pregnancies edema, high blood pressure, and proteinuria. Premature labor is a significant and common complication of multiple pregnancies. Statistically, about 60% of twins are born before their due date [27]. The risk is about three times more than in the case of normal twin pregnancies [28].

9.2 Twin-twin transfusion syndrome (TTTS)

Another thing you should remember when it comes to twins with IVF is the risk of TTTS. When two identical twins share the placenta, the possibility of twin-twin transfusion can occur at about 5%. Life-threatening conditions might happen if one of the babies had more blood than the other twins [29].

9.3 Intrauterine growth restriction (IUGR)

IUGR is a complication that might occur in multiple pregnancies. It means that one of the babies is not developing at the pace it should. Due to this delayed growth, several health implications are imminent for either or both babies [30].

9.4 Cesarean section

Carrying twins might also mean that a cesarean section might be the method of delivering twins having a higher incidence of cesarean section. Compared with vaginal birth, recovering from a cesarean section requires more time, and looking after two babies after a cesarean section can be very difficult [19]. Low birth weight and premature delivery, depending on the time of the delivery, heart problems, problems with breathing, hearing, vision, and cerebral palsy are all issues that may occur [31].

10. Conclusion

Multiple pregnancies have high maternal and neonatal complications, especially preterm delivery, which increases the risk of significant neonatal morbidity and mortality. Promotion of the elective single embryo transfer strategy is needed to reduce multiple pregnancies following IVF technologies.

Disclosure

I state that this introduction has not been previously published, nor being considered for publication elsewhere. No conflict of interest.

Author details

Hassan S. Abduljabbar
Dr. Erfan and Bagedo General Hospital and Jeddah Fertility Center, Jeddah, Saudi Arabia

*Address all correspondence to: profaj17@yahoo.com

References

[1] Beck JJ, Bruins S, Mbarek H, Davies GE, Boomsma DI. Biology and genetics of dizygotic and monozygotic twinning. In: Twin and Higher-Order Pregnancies. Cham: Springer; 2021. pp. 31-50

[2] Vitthala S, Gelbaya TA, Brison DR, Fitzgerald CT, Nardo LG. The risk of monozygotic twins after assisted reproductive technology: A systematic review and meta-analysis. Human Reproduction Update. 2009;**15**(1):45-55

[3] Umstad MP, Calais-Ferreira L, Scurrah KJ, Hall JG, Craig JM. Twins and twinning. Emery and Rimoin's Principles and Practice of Medical Genetics and Genomics. 2019;**3**:387-414

[4] Bhalotra S, Clarke D. Twin birth and maternal condition. Review of Economics and Statistics. 2019;**101**(5):853-864

[5] Tambiah SJ. Transnational movements, diaspora, and multiple modernities. In: Multiple Modernities. Vol. 1. Routledge; 29 Sep 2017. pp. 163-194. Available from: taylorfrancis.com

[6] Akinseye K, Anifowoshe A, Owolodun O, Aina O, Iyiola O. Frequency of twinning in Nigeria. A review. Manila Journal of Science. 2019;**12**:78-88

[7] Hotz C, Loechl C, de Brauw A, Eozenou P, Gilligan D, Moursi M, et al. A large-scale intervention to introduce orange sweet potato in rural Mozambique increases vitamin a intakes among children and women. British Journal of Nutrition. 2012;**108**(1):163-176

[8] Sobek A, Prochazka M, Klaskova E, Lubusky M, Pilka R. High incidence of monozygotic twinning in infertility treatment. Biomedical Papers. 2016;**160**(3):358-362

[9] Martin JA, Hamilton BE, Osterman MJ. Three decades of twin births in the United States, 1980-2009. NCHS Data Brief. Jan 2012;(80):1-8. PMID: 22617378

[10] Shelke PS, Jagtap PN. Twin pregnancy a complicating journey for both mothers and babies: Elaborate review. International Journal of Basic & Clinical Pharmacology. Mar 2020;**9**(4):674. DOI: 10.18203/2319-2003.ijbcp20201196

[11] Bókkon I, Vas JP, Császár N, Lukács T. Challenges to free will: Transgenerational epigenetic information, unconscious processes, and vanishing twin syndrome. Reviews in the Neurosciences. 2014;**25**(1):163-175

[12] Mogford K. development in twins. Language Development in Exceptional Circumstances. 2013:80

[13] Park SH, Lim DO. Distribution and definition of degree for inter twin birth weight discordance. Journal of Health Informatics and Statistics. 2019;**44**(3):286-291

[14] Bricker L. Optimal antenatal care for twin and triplet pregnancy: The evidence base. Best Practice & Research Clinical Obstetrics & Gynaecology. 2014;**28**(2):305-317

[15] Melka S, Miller J, Fox NS. Labor and delivery of twin pregnancies. Obstetrics and Gynecology Clinics. 2017;**44**(4):645-654

[16] Black M, Bhattacharya S. Epidemiology of multiple pregnancy and the effect of assisted conception. In: Seminars in Fetal and Neonatal Medicine. Vol. 15, No. 6. WB Saunders; 2010. pp. 306-312

[17] Adamson GD, Norman RJ. Why are multiple pregnancy rates and single embryo transfer rates so different globally, and what do we do about it? Fertility and Sterility. 2020;**114**(4):680-689

[18] Diamond MP, Mitwally M, Casper R, Ager J, Legro RS, Brzyski R, et al. Estimating rates of multiple gestation pregnancies: Sample size calculation from the assessment of multiple intrauterine gestations from ovarian stimulation (AMIGOS) trial. Contemporary Clinical Trials. 2011;**32**(6):902-908

[19] Young BC, Wylie BJ. Effects of twin gestation on maternal morbidity. In: Seminars in Perinatology. Vol. 36, No. 3. WB Saunders; 2012. pp. 162-168

[20] Chauhan SP, Scardo JA, Hayes E, Abuhamad AZ, Berghella V. Twins: Prevalence, problems, and preterm births. American journal of Obstetrics and Gynecology. 2010;**203**(4):305-315

[21] Fauser BC. Medical approaches to ovarian stimulation for infertility. In: Yen and Jaffe's Reproductive Endocrinology. Elsevier; 2019. pp. 743-778

[22] Pison G, Monden C, Smits J. Twinning rates in developed countries: Trends and explanations. Population and Development Review. 2015;**41**(4):629-649

[23] Kissin DM, Kulkarni AD, Mneimneh A, Warner L, Boulet SL, Crawford S, et al. Embryo transfer practices and multiple births resulting from assisted reproductive technology: An opportunity for prevention. Fertility and Sterility. 2015;**103**(4):954-961

[24] Pandian Z, Marjoribanks J, Ozturk O, Serour G, Bhattacharya S. Number of embryos for transfer following in vitro fertilisation or intra-cytoplasmic sperm injection. Cochrane Database of Systematic Reviews. 2013;(7):25

[25] Wen SW, Miao Q, Taljaard M, Lougheed J, Gaudet L, Davies M, et al. Associations of assisted reproductive technology and twin pregnancy with risk of congenital heart defects. JAMA Pediatrics. 2020;**174**(5):446-454

[26] Knopman JM, Krey LC, Oh C, Lee J, McCaffrey C, Noyes N. What makes them split? Identifying risk factors that lead to monozygotic twins after in vitro fertilization. Fertility and Sterility. 2014;**102**(1):82-89

[27] Phipps EA, Thadhani R, Benzing T, Karumanchi SA. Pre-eclampsia: Pathogenesis, novel diagnostics and therapies. Nature Reviews Nephrology. 2019;**15**(5): 275-289

[28] Vogel JP, Chawanpaiboon S, Moller AB, Watananirun K, Bonet M, Lumbiganon P. The global epidemiology of preterm birth. Best Practice & Research Clinical Obstetrics &Gynaecolog. 2018;**52**:3-12

[29] Simpson LL, Society for Maternal-Fetal Medicine (SMFM). Twin-twin transfusion syndrome. American journal of Obstetrics and Gynecology. 2013;**208**(1):3-18

[30] Valsky DV, Eixarch E, Martinez JM, Crispi F, Gratacós E. Selective intrauterine growth restriction in monochorionic twins: Pathophysiology, diagnostic approach and management dilemmas. In: Seminars in Fetal and Neonatal Medicine. Vol. 15, No. 6. WB Saunders; 2010. pp. 342-348

[31] Barzilay E, Mazaki-Tovi S, Amikam U, de Castro H, Haas J, Mazkereth R, et al. Mode of delivery of twin gestation with very low birthweight: Is vaginal delivery safe? American Journal of Obstetrics and Gynecology. 2015;**213**(2):219-2e1

Chapter 2

Multiple Pregnancy: Boon or Bane – An Indian Perspective

R. Kishore Kumar and B.R. Usha

Abstract

In the era of rising multiple pregnancy, it is important for us to analyse the recent trends. Assisted reproductive technology has brought hope to many childless couples. But it comes with a price. The prevalence of multiple gestation globally at present is 32 per 1000 deliveries. Recent studies from India report an incidence of 30.5 per 1000 deliveries. The most important complication associated with multiple gestation is prematurity. From the neonatology point of view, the increase in multiple gestation has opened an additional opportunity for the neonatologists to see and manage more preterm babies. Infants born after a multifetal pregnancy are associated with an increased risk of prematurity, cerebral palsy, learning disabilities, slow language development, behavioural difficulties, chronic lung disease, developmental delay, and death. The relative risk of cerebral palsy in twins and triplets compared to a singleton is 4.9 and 12.7, respectively. Foetal reduction as a routine should be discussed with all couples with multiple gestation including twins, to improve the pregnancy and neonatal outcome. Any multifetal gestation is a high-risk pregnancy should be managed efficiently by a multidisciplinary team involving Senior Obstetricians, neonatologists, intensivists, anaesthesiologists, physicians and nursing team in a well-equipped centre.

Keywords: multiple pregnancy, foetal reduction, prematurity

1. Introduction

In the era of rising multiple pregnancy, it is important for us to analyse the recent trends. This chapter will highlight the same and the recent updates in the management from an Indian perspective.

The prevalence of multiple gestation globally at present is 32 per 1000 deliveries [1]. Recent studies from India report an incidence of 30.5 per 1000 deliveries [2]. These again vary with respect to private and government sectors, with more spontaneous multiple pregnancies in the government and more ART (assisted reproductive technology)-associated multiple pregnancies seen in the private sector.

Due to the changes in lifestyle, delayed age of childbearing and stressful life, we see a lot of increase in infertility. At least one in five couples are known to have fertility issues these days. These ART techniques including ovulation induction with or without IUI are associated with a risk of multiple pregnancy of 8–10%. This increases up to 30% with IVF and two blastocyst transfer.

Assisted reproductive technology has brought hope to many childless couples. But it comes with a price. Each blastocyst of good quality can potentially give rise to four foetuses. There are many case reports of multiple pregnancy after a single-embryo transfer. With the routine trend of many ART specialists adopting two or more embryo transfer to achieve better pregnancy rates, the incidence of multiple gestation is known to increase.

From the neonatology point of view, the increase in multiple gestation has opened an additional challenge to the neonatologists to manage more preterm babies. Gone are those days, when extremely premature babies less than 28 weeks were not considered viable and were not resuscitated. Extremely premature babies with less as 24 weeks or 450 gm rate are being resuscitated and managed efficiently in NICU and successfully sent home. Perinatal outcomes may not be optimum with extremely premature babies, but over the last few decades, we have learnt a lot about extremely premature new-born care. This has helped us to analyse the data and improvise our protocols in the management.

2. Causes of multiple gestation

1. Higher maternal age

2. Family history of twinning

3. Prior OCPs use—the cycles immediately after stoppage of contraceptive pills will be associated with superovulation, higher fecundity and multiple pregnancy also

4. ART—ovulation induction carries a risk of multiple pregnancy of 8%. Incidence increases with IVF (*in vitro* fertilisation) and blastocyst transfer. Each blastocyst can potentially give rise to four foetuses in utero.

2.1 Types of multiple gestation

1. Dizygotic—resulting from fertilisation of two separate ova. They are fraternal twins and do not look alike. They are always dichorionic diamniotic.

2. Monozygotic—resulting from a single fertilised zygote. They look alike.

Depending on the timing of cell division after fertilisation, chorionicity and amnionicity develop in monozygotic twins. After fertilisation, when the division happens.

1. 0–4 days—dichorionic, diamniotic

2. 4–8 days—monochorionic, diamniotic

3. 8–12 days—monochorionic, monoamniotic

4. After 12 days—conjoined twins.

2.2 Multiple pregnancy boon or bane

It may be very nice to have twin babies, triplets might be fancy, and quadruplets would be a burden. But any multiple gestation is termed a high-risk pregnancy.

The most important complication associated with multiple gestation is prematurity (Kamlesh Kumari et al. [3]). 65.7% increased chances of preterm labour and 61.4% increased chances of having a caesarean section have been reported with multiple pregnancies – with most common reason being malpresentation of one of the fetuses.

2.3 Maternal complications

The maternal complications with multiple pregnancy include preterm labour, PPROM, anaemia, gestational hypertension, gestational diabetes, polyamnios, oligoamnios, haemorrhage including post-partum, and more incidence of caesarean delivery.

2.4 Foetal complications

Infants born after a multifetal pregnancy are associated with the increased risk of prematurity, cerebral palsy, learning disabilities, slow language development, behavioural difficulties, chronic lung disease, developmental delay, and death. The relative risk of cerebral palsy in twins and triplets compared to a singleton is 4.9 and 12.7, respectively.

Determination of chorionicity is very important in these pregnancies.

1. Dichorionic diamniotic pregnancies carry least complication rates. This is the most common variety.

2. Monochorionic twins are at higher risk of complications and among them monoamniotic are at the highest risk. The risk is due to placental vascular anastomoses and/or placental sharing. The complications include selective growth restriction, twin reverse arterial perfusion sequence (TRAP), twin-to-twin transfusion syndrome (TTTS), and twin anaemia-polycythemia sequence (TAPS).

The other complications include single foetal demise, congenital anomalies, discordant twins, conjoint twins, birth asphyxia, low birth weight, birth trauma, still birth, perinatal death and prolonged NICU stay. In India, 10% of the perinatal mortality can be attributed to twin pregnancies (**Table 1**).

The above comparison reports various descriptive Indian studies done in recent years with respect to multiple pregnancy. The mean age of women in these studies was in the range of 25–27 yrs. So, they are all young women mostly conceptions with ART. Preterm labour was the most common complication with incidence going up to 84.31%, and in them, preterm premature rupture of membranes was noted in up to 23.52%. Among the medical complications, anaemia was the most common complication ranging from 30.7 to 91.67%. This is due to nutritional deficiency developed due to increased demand of twins or triplets or due to hyperemesis associated with these pregnancies. Incidence of gestational diabetes is up to 13.73%, and gestational hypertension is seen up to 37.5%, which can be explained by a larger placenta seen in these pregnancies. Antepartum haemorrhage was seen in up to 5.95% patients. Most of these patients present with low-lying placenta mainly due to a larger placental surface and develop intermittent spotting

Study	Anita et al. [2]	Kamlesh et al. [3]	Nutan Yadav et al. [4]	P Upreti et al. [5]
Number of patients	51	70	72	218
Mean age		27.6	26.08	25.4
Preterm labour	84.31%	25.4%	79.2%	58.3%
PPROM	23.53%	18.3%	22.29%	4.1%
Gestational diabetes	13.73%	5.6%	2.7%	
Gestational HTN	15.68%	22.5%	37.5%	21.1%
Anaemia	62.74%	26.8%	91.67%	30.7%
APH	3.33	1.4%	2.7%	5.95
Malpresentation	47%	37.8	22.2%	36.9%
Caesarean	58.82%	64.3	50%	49%
Anomalies	0.97%	0		
Foetal demise	1.94	0		
Perinatal mortality	17.48%	12.9		
IUGR	14.56%	11.4%	20.8%	
Growth discordance		21.4%		25%
NICU admission	20.38%			

Table 1.
Demographics of multiple gestation studies in India.

or bleeding creating panic in patients. Many of them also develop abruption associated with hypertension. There is an increased incidence of postpartum haemorrhage also in multiple gestation mainly due to overdistended uterus and post-partum atony. It would be wise to be prepared for it with active management of the third stage of labour and keeping blood and blood products cross-matched and ready.

Caesarean delivery is the most common of delivery in multiple pregnancy seen in up to 64.3% mainly due to malpresentation (in up to 47%). Normal delivery is an option only in twin deliveries and not on triplets or higher orders. In twins, cephalic-cephalic position is the most common presentation where vaginal delivery is feasible. The second most common is cephalic and second breech position where vaginal delivery also can be done. However, in these cases, there is a small risk of the requirement of Caesarean for second twin due to malpresentation or non-progress of labour. In cases of transverse lie or both breech or other presentations, Caesarean would be the option. In the breech and second cephalic presentation, there is risk of the first twin's head getting locked against the second twin (interlocking twin) and hence vaginal deliveries should be thought about only when the first twin is in cephalic presentation.

3. Foetal reduction

It has been developed since the 1980s, as a method to reduce the multiple gestation to twin or singleton gestation to reduce the complications. It involves preliminary screening of foetuses at NT scan and reduction of foetuses that are abnormal or relatively abnormal. If there are no abnormal foetuses, then a decision is taken based on the most accessible foetus for the procedure. Gender selection is not allowed in India as per PCPNDT rules and hence shall not be a criterion to decide. It is done as a day-care procedure with some minimal local anaesthesia. It involves transabdominal ultrasound-guided injection of KCl into the foetal heart to stop its function. Some studies report doing chorionic villus sampling of foetuses and FISH before reduction. The procedure is ideally done between 12 and 14 weeks after the NT scan to allow for spontaneous reductions to happen till then and NT screening to be done. In up to 20 to 60%, spontaneous reduction to singleton pregnancy happens [6]. The demised twin disappears as a vanishing twin. There has been an increasing trend of reducing even twins to singleton to avoid the complications associated with multiple births.

Jung Ryeol Lee et al. [7] report early foetal reduction at 6–8 weeks by transvaginal ultrasound guidance using a 19G needle. Cardiac puncture and amniotic fluid aspiration is done to produce foetal reduction, which may be added on with KCl injection. However, this study reports better pregnancy and foetal outcomes with early foetal reduction at 6–8weeks without using KCl.

The foetal reduction procedure is therefore not limited to triplets or quadruplet gestations. Twin gestation reduced to singleton, do better according to studies. We do see patients refusing reduction on moral or religious grounds, thinking about foeticide or about the risk of miscarriage.

The procedure is associated with a small risk of miscarriage and infection, which should be explained to the couple against the risks involved in continuing with the multiple gestation.

Foetal reduction as a routine should be discussed with all couples with multiple gestation, including twins to improve the pregnancy and the neonatal outcome. This counselling should involve an explanation of the risks specifically with multiple pregnancy and the option to reduce the pregnancy. The moral and ethical background should be kept in mind before counselling the couple about the procedure.

4. Interventions to reduce multiple gestation

1. Routine single-embryo transfer—many European countries have adopted routine single-embryo transfer to avoid multiple gestation. In such countries, healthcare and IVF treatment are government funded and multiple IVF cycles are also funded by the government. So, the patient is not concerned about the reduced pregnancy rates with single-embryo transfer against double-embryo transfer. However, in India, where all infertility treatments are neither covered under insurance nor are government funded and when the patient has to spend out of his pocket, it becomes difficult for them to accept any method with slightly reduced pregnancy rates. Hence, it becomes difficult for Indian clinicians to convince patients for single-embryo transfer.

2. Cancelling ovulation induction when multiple follicles are developed—sometimes when we give ovulation-inducing agents to patients either letrozole, clomiphene citrate, or gonadotrophins, we do see some patients hyper-responding with the development of more than three mature follicles. It would be a wise decision to not give ovulation trigger or human chorionic gonadotropin injection in cases where more than three mature follicles have developed. In that way, multiple pregnancies can be avoided.

3. Efficient counselling of the couple to make an informed choice—we are in an era where patients are bombarded with information all over. It is essential for them to make to understand the risks and complications associated with multiple pregnancy and the future outcome and with that perspective, the concept of foetal reduction.

4. Offer foetal reduction to all multiple gestations including twins. Infants born after a multifetal pregnancy including twins are associated with the increased risk of prematurity, cerebral palsy, learning disabilities, slow language development, behavioural difficulties, chronic lung disease, developmental delay, and death. Considering the perinatal morbidity and NICU care requirement in these twin gestations, it would be prudent to give all couples an option to consider about foetal reduction of twins to the singleton.

5. Antenatal care

It is important to determine the chorionicity with a good transvaginal ultrasound at the time of the dating scan (7–10 weeks). According to the chorionicity, the pregnancy is categorised, and the antenatal visit schedule is planned. All women should be offered screening for trisomy 21 at 11–13 + 6 weeks of gestation. This ultrasound can be combined with first-trimester biochemistry (serum PAPP-A and beta-Hcg) to make it combined screening with the better detection rates. For triplets or higher-order pregnancies, only nuchal translucency screening should be done.

The next level of ultrasound screening is an anomaly scan, which is offered between 18 and 22 weeks. Monochorionic pregnancies should be scanned at 16–17, 19–20, and 21–22 weeks. Monoamniotic twins should be screened from 15 to 16 weeks and 18 to 20 weeks. A five-chamber view of the heart should be carried out at 18–19 weeks and 21–22 weeks. Further growth scan shall include complete documentation of full biometry, foetal weight, liquor, and bladder size. Scans should be performed at a frequency dictated by the chorionicity (**Table 2**) [8].

It is important for the obstetrician to be well versed with the complications associated with multiple gestation. Accordingly, the antenatal visits should be scheduled, and the pregnancy closely monitored. Where required, a multidisciplinary team involving foetal medicine consultants, neonatologists and physicians should be involved in the management. Routine antenatal visits should include screening for anaemia, hypertension, diabetes, and foetal heartbeat assessment.

5.1 Cervical length screening

It is done by transvaginal ultrasound at 12 weeks, 16 weeks, 20 weeks and 24 weeks. Cervical length less than 2.5 cm is considered short. Prophylactic cervical cerclage in multiple gestation is controversial. Evidence suggests that cervical length is a moderate predictor of spontaneous preterm labour in twin pregnancy. Vaginal progesterone may reduce this risk in women with a twin pregnancy. However, in patients with ART conception especially with polycystic ovaries that are known to be associated with cervical insufficiency, prophylactic cervical cerclage would be beneficial. It is ideally applied after NT scan between 13 and 14 weeks or if history indicated, at least 2 weeks before the previous miscarriage.

Type of pregnancy	Growth scans
Dichorionic gestation	24, 28, 32, 36
Monochorionic	24, 28, 32, 34
Mono amniotic	24,26, 28, 32, 34
Triplet/quadruplet	Individualised

Table 2.
Suggested ultrasound scans for multiple gestation pregnancies.

5.2 Antenatal corticosteroids

If elective delivery or Caesarean is planned before 38 weeks, antenatal corticosteroids are warranted to be given, either betamethasone or dexamethasone. This is according to the present data available. A lot of newer studies are ongoing with respect to the assessment of newborn adverse effects due to antenatal steroids. The present protocols suggest two doses of betamethasone, 12 mg given intramuscular, 24 hrs apart. Similarly, dexamethasone can be given 6 mg, 12th hourly four doses 6 hrs apart.

5.3 Antenatal magnesium sulphate

BEAM trial [9] in 2002 first proposed the beneficial effects of antenatal magnesium sulphate in women at imminent preterm delivery. All pregnancies that are at risk of premature delivery shall be given an intravenous infusion of magnesium sulphate over 24 hrs. It is given as a loading dose of 4 g slow IV over 5 minutes followed by 1 g/hour infusion for 24 hrs. Magnesium sulphate is a weak tocolytic. It is very efficient in preventing cerebral palsy in preterm newborns (RR 0.70, 95% CI 0.55–0.89). It also has a neuroprotective role in preventing intra-ventricular haemorrhage.

5.4 Tocolysis

Preterm labour being the most common complication with multiple pregnancy, it is essential to provide tocolysis to the patient at least to have antenatal steroid cover for 48 hrs. This would improve neonatal neurological and respiratory outcomes. The most effective tocolysis available is Atosiban, which is an oxytocin antagonist and should be the first choice of drug. It is started as a 0.9 ml (6.75MG) loading dose intravenous and followed by a high-dose infusion of 300 mcg per minute for 3 hrs. This is followed by a low-dose maintenance infusion of 100 mcg per minute for the next 45 hrs. The total dose infused shall not exceed 330.75 mg. The second-best drug for tocolysis is nifedipine given as a loading dose of 30–40 mg followed by 10 mg sixth hourly. Nifedipine being a calcium channel blocker relaxes the smooth muscle of the uterus and induces tocolysis. The main aim of tocolysis is to safely transfer the mother to a tertiary care centre well equipped for multiple gestation and preterm newborn care and also to allow for the antenatal steroid prophylaxis to act. Hence, it should not be prolonged for more than 48 hrs. Tocolysis should be weighed against the maternal risks of sepsis and pulmonary oedema before continuing the therapy.

6. Delivery plan

It is essential to have institutional deliveries for all multiple pregnancies. The centre should be well equipped for emergency Caesarean facilities, blood bank, tertiary NICU care, and a multidisciplinary team involving intensivists, physicians, endocrinologists, and foetal medicine consultants. The timing of delivery is crucial to optimise the neonatal outcomes. The mode of delivery again should be individualised, and the main deciding factor is the foetal presentation (**Table 3**).

6.1 Intrapartum monitoring

Monitoring twin foetuses in labour can be difficult at times. They should be monitored with twin foetal heart probes to avoid the same foetal heart being traced twice on cardiotocography. Always perform a portable ultrasound bedside to ascertain the presentation at the start of labour.

6.2 Post-partum period

There is more incidence of post-partum haemorrhage in these women, mainly due to an overdistended uterus in pregnancy. The obstetric team should be prepared with oxytocics, blood and blood products at the time of delivery to efficiently manage it. Active management of the third stage of labour should be routinely done in all women to reduce the incidence of haemorrhage.

6.3 Breastfeeding

It can be a challenge with respect to demand in twin and triplets gestation. Most of these babies are born prematurely with poor suckling or latching, and hence, there can be difficult establishing the feeding. More so many of these babies stay in the NICU in the initial few days or weeks when rooming in and breastfeeding could be difficult to establish. As suckling is the most important stimulus for further breast milk production, when the baby is away from the mother breastfeeding establishment becomes a challenge. Feeding both babies simultaneously is another technique to increase the milk output in the mother.

Type of multiple pregnancies	Planned birth to be offered at	Increased risk of foetal death beyond	Mode of delivery
Dichorionic diamniotic	37 weeks	37 + 6weeks	Individualised
Monochorionic diamniotic	36 weeks	36 + 6	Individualised
Monochorionic monoamniotic	32 to 33 + 6 weeks	33 + 6	Caesarean
Trichorionic triamniotic	35 weeks	35 + 6	Caesarean
Dichorionic triamniotic	35 weeks	35 + 6	Caesarean

Table reference [8].

Table 3.
Recommended time table for delivery of multiple pregnancies.

7. Conclusion

Multiple pregnancy is a high-risk pregnancy to be always managed by an efficient and experienced multidisciplinary team. Foetal reduction is an option to be explained to all couples with multiple pregnancy to reduce the neonatal and childhood morbidity. Foetal reduction is more common in LMIC countries than in developed world because of the higher morbidity and cost of healthcare associated with multiple pregnancies.

Author details

R. Kishore Kumar[1,2]* and B.R. Usha[3]

1 Senior Consultant Neonatologist and Paediatrician, Cloudnine Hospitals, Bangalore, India

2 Adjunct Professor in Neonatology and Paediatrics, Notre Dame University, Perth, Australia

3 Consultant Obstetrician, Gynaecologist and Laparoscopic Surgeon Cloudnine Hospitals, Jayanagar, Bangalore, India

*Address all correspondence to: drkishore@cloudninecare.com

References

[1] El-Toukhy T, Bhattacharya S, Akande V. A on behalf of the Royal College of Obstetricians and Gynaecologists. Multiple pregnancies following assisted conception. Scientific Impact Paper No. 22. BJOG. 2018

[2] Madan A, Meena JKS, Puri A. Maternal and fetal outcome in multiple pregnancy. International Journal of Health and Clinical Research. 2020;**3**(12):221-226

[3] Kumari K, Mishra M, Jhanwar A, Kumari A. Fetomaternal outcome in twin pregnancies: A retrospective analysis from a tertiary care centre. Journal of Clinical and Diagnostic Research. 2020;**14**(7):QC01-QC05

[4] Yadav N, Alwani M, Singh A. Incidence and perinatal outcome of multiple pregnancy in a tertiary care centre in Central India. International Journal of Reproduction, Contraception, Obstetrics and Gynecology. 2018;7(5):1912-1917

[5] Upreti P. Twin pregnancies: Incidence and outcomes in a tertiary health centre of Uttarakhand, India. International Journal of Reproduction, Contraception, Obstetrics and Gynecology. 2018;7(9):3520-3525

[6] Beriwal S, Impey L, Ioannou C. Multifetal pregnancy reduction and selective termination. The Obstetrician & Gynaecologist. 2020;**22**:284-292. Available from: https://obgyn.onlinelibrary.wiley.com/doi/10.1111/tog.12690

[7] Lee JR, Ku S-Y, Jee BC, Suh CS, Kim KC, Kim SH. Pregnancy outcomes of different methods for multifetal pregnancy reduction: A comparative study. Journal of Korean Medical Science 2008;**23**:111-116. The Korean Academy ISSN 1011-8934 of Medical Sciences. DOI: 10.3346/jkms.2008.23.1.111

[8] Antenatal management of multiple pregnancies: NICE guidelines. March 2013

[9] Rouse, Dwight. Beneficial effects of antenatal magnesium sulfate (BEAM Trial)

Chapter 3

Types of Multiple Pregnancy

Tshililo Mashamba

Abstract

Multiple pregnancy is condition where more than one offsprings are formed. This result from either fertilization of more than one ovum individually by separate sperms or division of fertilized ovum. The implantation sites may be in different part of the genital organs and even the peritoneal cavity. The physiology of monozygotic multiple pregnancy is not fully understood as the trigger has not yet been identified. The incidence of multiple pregnancy is increasing, and this is as a result of assisted reproductive technologies.

Keywords: multiple pregnancy, dichorionic, monochorionic, twin, heretopic

1. Introduction

Multiple pregnancy refers to a pregnancy with more than one embryo. The embryos may grow in the same uterine pregnancy as a result of either two or three separate ova were fertilized or one ovum fertilized, and the embryo divided two or more embryos developed. Where two or more ova are fertilized individually the resultant pregnancy is called dizygous if two ova were fertilized and multizygous multiple pregnancy if three or more ova were fertilized. The implantation site also determines the naming of the type of multiple pregnancy. The dizygous or multizygous multiple pregnancies result in each embryo having its own placenta and amniotic sac and are independent of each other. Where one ovum is fertilized, and the embryo divides it is called monozygous multiple pregnancy. Zygosity is the degree of identity in the genome.

The incidence of multiple pregnancy is increasing as a result of increasing use of assisted reproductive technology [1, 2]. Twin pregnancy account for 2–4% of the total number of births. Spontaneous twin pregnancy rates vary worldwide [3]. The incidence of higher order multiple pregnancy is not fully reported but there are lot of case reports noted. The incidence of triplet pregnancies has been estimated to be one in thousand pregnancies [4]. Different types of multiple pregnancy will be discussed.

2. Dizygous multiple pregnancy

Dizygotic multiple pregnancy is derived from fertilization of two ova by two sperms and they may be of same sex or different sex. Their genetic composition is different because it comes from different ova and different sperms. These are just two siblings in the same patient. Dizygotic multiple pregnancy contributes two thirds of all multiple pregnancies. The implantation may be at the same site or different sites. Each of the embryo has its own chorion (placenta) and amniotic membrane as in **Figure 1**. They are also called fraternal multiple pregnancy [5]. Fertilization may occur during the same sexual activity or different sexual activities during the same

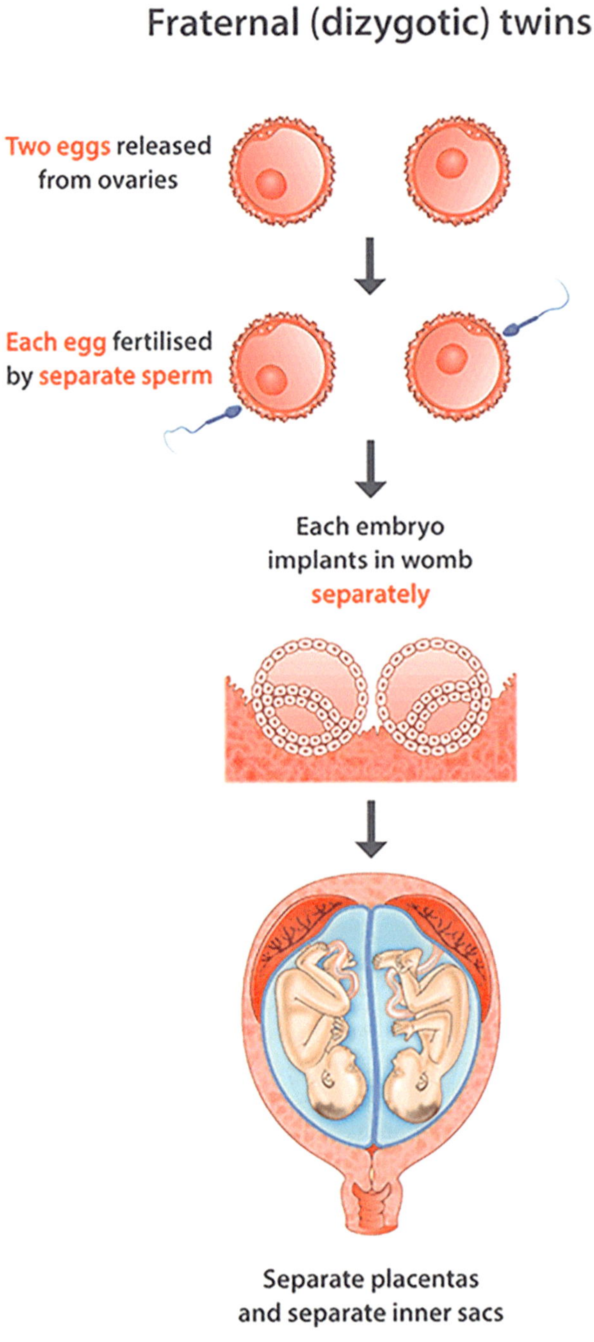

Figure 1.
Site of implantation of dizygotic multiple pregnancy.

One fetus	singleton
Two fetuses	Twins
Three fetuses	Triplets
Four fetuses	Quadruplets
Five fetuses	Quintuplets
Six fetuses	Sextuplets
Seven fetuses	Septuplets
Eight fetuses	Octuplets
Nine fetuses	Nonuplets
Ten fetuses	decuplets

Table 1.
Subtypes of multiple pregnancy.

menstrual cycle. Fertilization of the second ovum during different sexual exposure is called superfecundation. This means that fertilization of the ovum when there is an existing early embryo. If fertilization of the second ovum and implantation occurs in subsequent menstrual cycle, this is superfetation. Upregulation of hypothalamic-pituitary-ovarian axis by luteal progesterone and then placental progesterone in the first trimester of pregnancy suppresses ovulation and makes the possibilities of superfetation unlikely [5, 6]. The physiology of superfetation is not well understood.

3. Intra uterine dizygotic multiple pregnancy

Implantation of all the embryos inside the endometrial cavity. This is the most common type of all multiple pregnancies. There may be two or more fetuses. The naming of the subtype depends on the number of fetuses (see **Table 1**).

4. Dicavitary multiple pregnancy

This is a type of multiple pregnancy occurring in a woman with embryological developmental malformation of the Mullerian or Wolffian ducts, characterized by complete failure of Mullerian ducts to fuse, resulting in two separate uterine cavities and cervices (**Figures 2** and **3**). There may associated vaginal anomalies like septum which may be longitudinal or transverse [7]. The anomalies may of different degrees with either fully developed or under developed and each with separate fallopian tube and endometrial cavity [8, 9]. Both uterine horns achieve a pregnancy at the same time when double ovulation has taken place (**Figure 4**). This only follows dizygotic multiple pregnancy and not possible with monozygotic pregnancy.

5. Heterotopic pregnancy

This refers to the occurrence of two pregnancies in different implantation sites simultaneously, mostly manifested as intrauterine and ectopic pregnancies 9ampullary in 80%). Heterotopic pregnancy is rare and estimated to occur in about 1 per

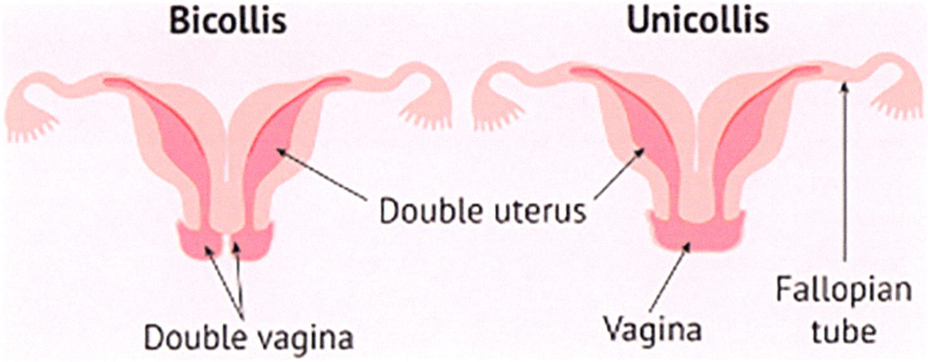

Figure 2.
Uterine didelphus.

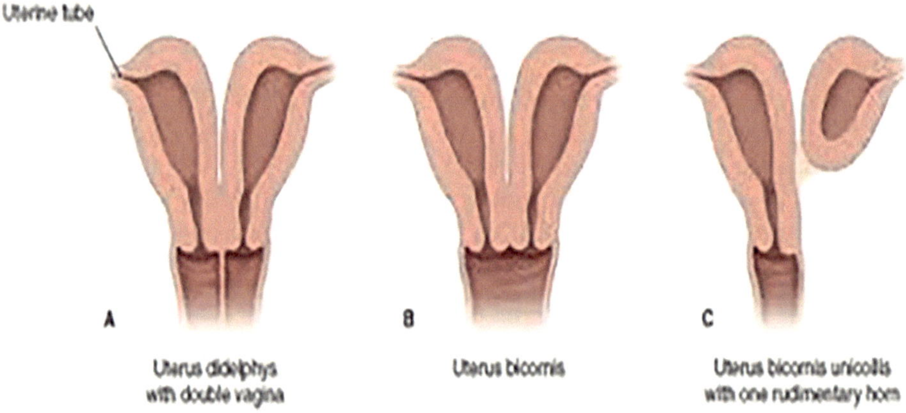

Figure 3.
Uterine anomaly.

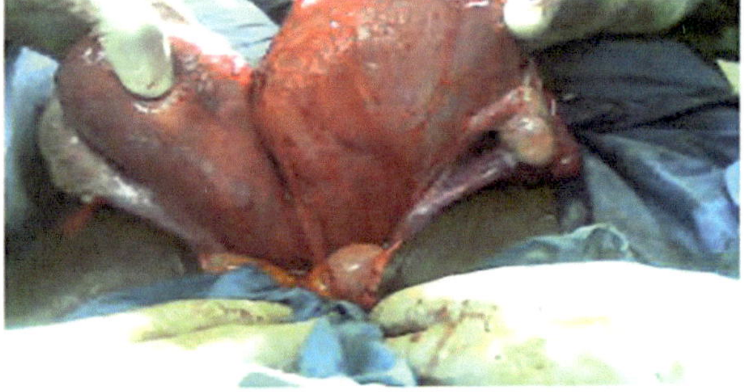

Figure 4.
Pregnancy on each uterus.

30,000 (0.006%–0.001%) spontaneous pregnancies while a higher prevalence may occur in assisted reproductive techniques that may reach up to 1 case per 100 cases (1–3%) (**Figure 5**) [10, 11].

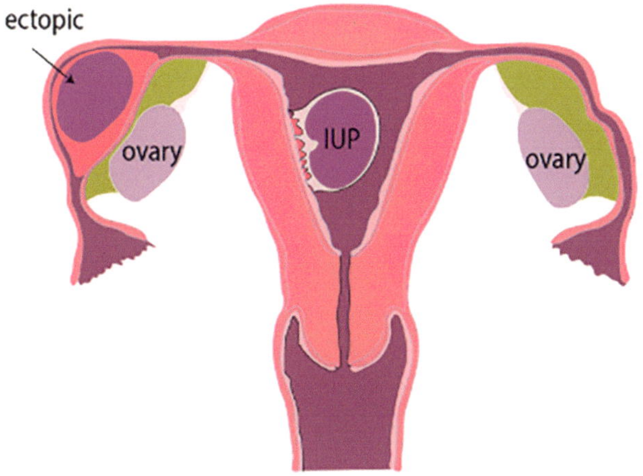

Figure 5.
Heterotopic oregnancy.

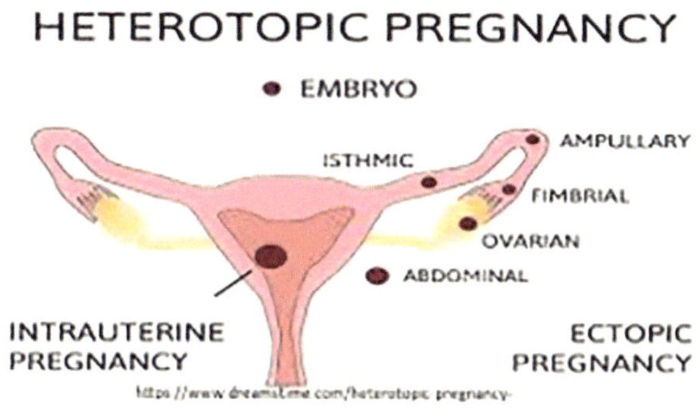

Figure 6.
Different sites for heterotopic pregnancy.

Another rare combination of heterotopic pregnancy is a combination of intrauterine and ovarian [12]. The occurrence of an ovarian heterotopic pregnancy is a singular event as it comprises only 2.35 of all heterotopic pregnancies. However, in the last decade there has been a significant increase of ectopic pregnancy and subsequent increase in heterotopic pregnancy. This increase has been attributed to higher incidence of pelvic inflammatory disease and the extended use of assisted reproductive technologies [12]. The implantation outside the endometrial cavity can be anywhere including any part of the fallopian tube, ovary and any part of peritoneal cavity as indicated on **Figure 6**.

6. Twin ectopic pregnancy

In ectopic pregnancy, the implantation occurs outside the uterine cavity post fertilization, either in singleton or multi-gestational ectopic pregnancy. The incidence of twin ectopic pregnancies is quite rare and is estimated to be 1 in 125,000

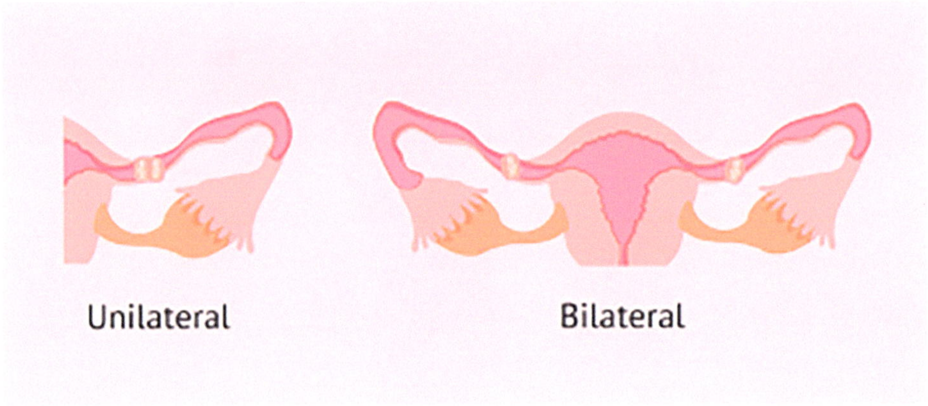

Figure 7.
Twin ectopic pregnancy.

pregnancies and that of twin tubal pregnancies to be 1 in 200 ectopic pregnancies (**Figure** 7) [13–15].

7. Monozygotic multiple pregnancy

Monozygotic (MZ) twins, also called identical twins, occur when a single egg cell is fertilized by a single sperm cell. The resulting zygote splits into two very early in development, leading to the formation of two separate embryos. MZ twins occur in 3–4 per 1000 births worldwide. Research suggests that most cases of MZ twinning are not caused by genetic factors. However, a few families with a larger-than-expected number of MZ twins have been reported, which indicates that genetics may play a role. It is possible that genes involved in sticking cells together (cell adhesion) may contribute to MZ twinning, although this hypothesis has not been confirmed. Most of the time, the cause of MZ twinning is unknown [16].

The theory proposes that monozygotic twin are formed when the blastocyst contains two inner cell masses, each of which lead to a separate fetus rather than by the embryo splitting while hatching from the zona pellucida. Monozygotic twins may be created artificially by embryo splitting. Monozygotic twins are genetically nearly identical and are always of the same sex unless there has been a mutation during development [16]. The timing of the division determines the chorionicity and amnionicity. Chorionicity refers to the placenta and amnionicity to amniotic sac on whether they are shared by the twins or not as indicated on **Figure 8**.

When the division occurs within 3 days of fertilization, a dichorionic twin pregnancy results, when the division occurs between 4 and 8 days a monochorionic diamniotic twin pregnancy develops and when division occurs from day 8 until day 12 or 13 the monochorionic mono amniotic twin pregnancy develops. After day 13 the division leads to conjoined twins. All this means is that the placenta is determined within 3 days otherwise no further division could take place after this period in regard to the placenta. Amniotic sac is determined between day 4 and day 8 after fertilization and complete fetal division within 12–13 days [17].

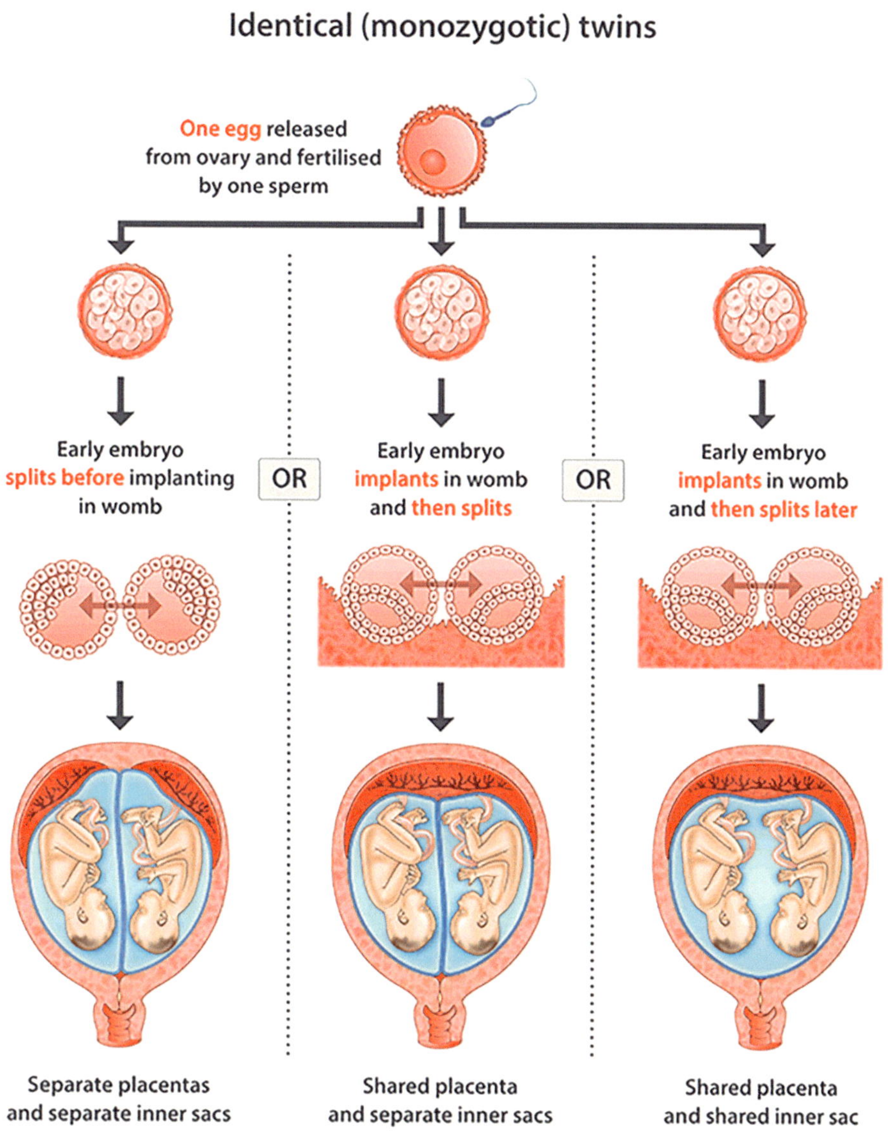

Figure 8.
Dichorionic diamniotic multiple pregnancy from monozygotic twins.

Monozygotic multiple pregnancies are not genetically inherited. The twinning is random, due to the splitting of the embryo, so all parents have equal chance of conceiving these types of twins [18]. The rate of monozygotic twins is 2,25 times higher in assisted conceptions than natural conceptions. Monozygotic twins have a chorionicity that relates to how early the fertilized egg divides. Of the live born twins 70–75% are monochorionic diamniotic, 25–30% are dichorionic diamniotic and 1% are monochorionic monoamniotic [19, 20].

Division of the fertilized ovum occurs within 3 days. Placental development is independent of each other, though genetic material is identical. This constitutes 25 to 30 percent of monozygotic twins [19].

8. Monochorionic diamniotic multiple pregnancy

This is the commonest type of twin pregnancy arising from monozygotic multiple pregnancy as its occurrence is 70–75%. The fetuses share a placenta but have different amniotic sacs. The division takes place between 4 and 8 days after fertilization. Overall 1 in 3 spontaneous twins or 1 in 300 pregnancies become monochorioninic diamniotic.

9. Monochorionic monoamniotic twins

This is the least common type of multiple pregnancies as it is just around 1% of all monochorionic multiple pregnancies. This type of multiple pregnancy is associated the highest rate of congenital anomalies starting with vascular malformation to conjoined twins.

10. Conclusion

Multiple pregnancy refers to conception with more than one embryo. There are different types of multiple pregnancy depending on the site of implantation and the number of embryos. Multiple pregnancy can develop from fertilization of more than one embryo (dizygotic) or from division of a single fertilized embryo (monozygotic). Dizygotic embryos have different genetic makeup while monozygotic embryos have almost the same genetic makeup unless mutation has taken place during development. Dizygotic multiple pregnancy is more common than monozygotic pregnancies because of assisted reproductive technology. The division of the embryo is guided by the time of division to achieve a particular type of monozygotic multiple pregnancy. Monochorionic multiple pregnancy is the commonest type of monozygotic multiple pregnancy compared to dichorionic and monoamniotic types.

Author details

Tshililo Mashamba
Department of Obstetrics and Gynaecology, Sefako Makgatho University Pretoria, South Africa

*Address all correspondence to: tjmashamba@yahoo.com

References

[1] Yayla M, Baytur Y. Multicentric multiple pregnancy study 1-Epidemiology. Perinatal Journal. 2008;**16**

[2] Mackie F, Morris R. Multiple gestation: Biology and epidemiology. Global Library Women. 2016;**40**:1756-2228

[3] Santana DS, Surita FG, Cecatti JG. Multiple pregnancy: Epidemiology and association with maternal and perinatal morbidity. Revista Brasileria de Ginecologia Obstetricia. 2018;**40**:554-562

[4] Smith LK, Manktelow BN, Draper ES, et al. Trends in the incidence and mortality of multiple births by socioeconomic deprivation and maternal age in England: Population-based cohort study. BMJ Open. 2014;**4**:e004514. DOI: 10.1136/bmjopen-2013-004514

[5] Painter JN, Hall JG. Twins and twinning. In: Emery and Rimoin's Principles and Practice of Medical Genetics. 2013

[6] Umstad MP, Craig JM. Superfetaion. In: Emery and Rimoin's Principles and Practice of Medical Genetics. 2019

[7] Al Yaqoubi HN, Fatema N. Successful vaginal delivery of naturally conceived dicavitary twin in didelphus uterus: A rare reported case. Hindawi Case Reports in Obstetrics and Gynecology. 2017

[8] Doruk A, Gozukara I, Burkaş G, Bilik E, Dilek TUK. Spontaneous twin pregnancy in uterus bicornis unicollis. Case Reports in Obstetrics and Gynecology. 2013;**2013**:3. Article ID: 834952

[9] Ilyas M, Dar M, Rafiq S, Khan I. Twin pregnancy in bicornuate uterus-one fetus in each horn. Journal of Fetal Medicine. 2018;**5**. DOI: 10.1007/s40556-018-0156-4

[10] Ali T, Tawab MA, ElHariri MAG, Ayad AA. Hetrotopic pregnancy: A case report. Egyptian Journal of Radiology and Nuclear Medicine. 2020;**51**:214

[11] Nabi U, Yousaf A, Ghaffar F, Salid S, Ahmed MMH. Heterotopic pregnancy—A diagnostic challenge. Six case reports and literature review. Cureus. 2019;**11**:11

[12] Basile F, Cesare DC, Quagliozzi L, Donati L, Bracaglia M, Caruso A, et al. Spontaneous heterotopic pregnancy simultaneous ovarian and intrauterine: A case report. Case Reports in Obstetrics and Gynecology. 2012. Article ID: 509694

[13] Madaan S, Jaiswal A, Banode P, Dhok A, Dewani D. Spontaneous twin ectopic pregnancy managed successfully with methotrexate-mediated ultrasound guided fetal reduction: A fertility-preserving approach. Cureus. 2021;**13**(8)

[14] Rolle CJ, Wai CY, Bawdon R, Santos-Ramos R, Hoffman B. Unilateral twin ectopic pregnancy in a patient with a history of multiple sexual transmitted infections. Infectious Diseases in Obstetrics and Gynecology. 2006:1-3

[15] Seak CJU, Goh ZNL, Wong AC, Seak JCY, Seak CK. Unilateral live twin tubal ectopic pregnancy presenting at 12 weeks of gestation. Medicine. 2019;**98**:38

[16] Available from: https://en.wikipedia.org/wiki/Twin

[17] Chitkara U, Berkowitz RL. Multiple Gestations, Obstetrics, Normal and Problem Pregnancies. 4th ed. 2002

[18] de Bellefonds C. Are Twins Hereditary? 2021. Retrieved from:

https://www.whattoexpect.com/pregnancy/twins-and-multiples/do-twins-really-run-in-families/

[19] Visintin C, Mugglestone MA, James D, Kilby MD, Guideline Development Group. Antenatal care for twin and triplet pregnancies: Summary of NICE guidance. BMJ (Clinical Research ed.). 2011;**343**:d5714. DOI: 10.1136/bmj.d5714

[20] Robinson J, Peat B, Dodd J, Atkinson E. South Australian Perinatal Practice Guideline: Twin pregnancy. 5th ed. 2014

Chapter 4

Multiple Gestation

Mandefro Yilma Asfaw

Abstract

Multiple pregnancies mean when the woman carries more than one fetus at a time. Multiple pregnancy, multiple gestation, and multifetal pregnancy are synonyms. These can be twins, triplets, quadruplets, or more. These types of pregnancy have become one of the most common high-risk pregnancies encountered by obstetricians. It is associated with an increased risk of both maternal and perinatal morbidity and mortality. The incidence of multiple pregnancies has risen significantly over the last four decades, primarily due to increased use of ovulation induction drugs. The symptoms and signs of multiple pregnancies include excessive nausea and vomiting, larger uterus than expected for the date of pregnancy, and excessive weight gain. The aim of this chapter is to discuss the occurrence, causes, epidemiology, maternal and perinatal morbidity and mortality, antepartum, and intrapartum management of multiple pregnancies.

Keywords: multiple pregnancy, chorionicity, zygosity, antenatal care, morbidity, mortality

1. Introduction

Multiple pregnancies are the presence of more than one fetus at a time. Simultaneous development of two fetuses, three fetuses, and four fetuses is called as twins, triplets, quadruplets, respectively, and so on. These types of pregnancies may result from two or more fertilization or from single fertilization followed by cleavage of the zygote or combination of both [1]. Such pregnancies are associated with increased maternal and perinatal morbidity and mortality compared to that singleton gestations. They can cause almost every potential complication of pregnancy except post-term delivery and macrosomia [2, 3]. Twins' pregnancy is the most common variety of multiple pregnancies and the rate of occurrence of multiple pregnancies decreases with an increased number of fetuses [4]. The rate and the number of both twin and higher-order multi-fetal births have increased dramatically over the last four decades, mainly due to ovulation induction and early detection by ultrasound [1, 5]. According to Hellin's rules, the mathematical frequency of multiple births is 1 in 80 $^{(n-1)}$ pregnancies, where n is the number of fetuses [4]. For example, twins 1 in 80 pregnancies, triplets 1 in 6400, quadruplets 1 in 512,000, etc. [4, 5].

2. Zygosity and chorionicty

Zygosity refers to the genetic makeup of the twin pregnancy while chorionicty indicates the placenta's membrane status [4]. Early determination of chorionicity is essential because it is a major factor in determining obstetrical risks, management, and outcomes [2, 3].

Twins can be either monozygotic or dizygotic.

- **Dizygotic (DZ) or fraternal twins** result from fertilization of two ova by two sperms during a single ovarian cycle.

- **Monozygotic (MZ) or identical twins** are the result of fertilization of a single ovum by single sperm and followed by splitting of the zygote. Chorionicity will depend on the timing of the division of the embryo. The following possibilities may occur:

    I. If the division takes place within 72 hours after fertilization, the resulting embryos will have two separate placenta, chorions, and amnions, that is, a thick four-layered intervening membrane. It accounts for 25 to 30% of MZ twins.

    II. If the division takes place between the 4th and 8th days of fertilization when the chorion is already formed, monochorionic, diamniotic twins will evolve with a thin two-layer dividing membrane. It accounts 70–75% of MZ twins.

    III. If the division occurs between 8th and 12th days of fertilization, the result will be a monochorionic and monoamniotic twin. It accounts 1–2% of MZ twins.

    IV. If the division occurs after 13th day of fertilization, the result will be a monochorionic, monoamniotic, and conjoined twins. It is a rare type of MZ and occurs in less than 1%.

The following table shows the relationship between the timing of division and the nature of membranes in twin pregnancy.

Time of cleavage	Nature of membranes
0–72 hours	Dichorionic, diamniotic
4–8 days	Monochorionic, diamniotic
9–12 days	Monochorionic, monoamniotic
After 13 days	Monochorionic, monoamniotic (conjoined twins)

The following figures show placentation in twin pregnancies [2].

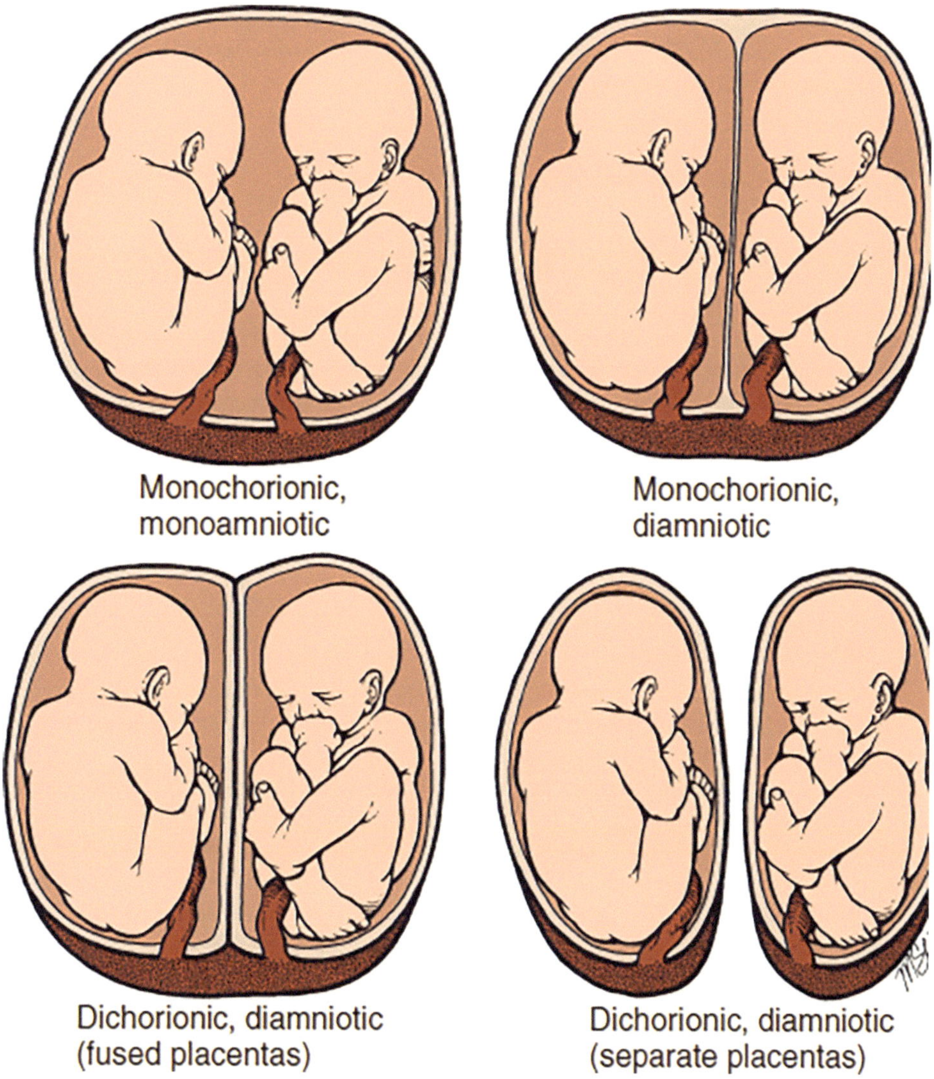

3. Rates and causes of monozygotic and dizygotic twinning

Dizygotic twins occur in about 1% to 1.5% and monozygotic twins 1 in 250 pregnancies among natural conception [2]. The rates of spontaneous DZ twinning are influenced by maternal age, family history, and race [2, 3, 6]. The frequency of MZ twinning is constant in all populations studied at about 1 in 250 births [3].

The risk for DZ twinning increases with maternal age, peaking at 37 years of age. Maternal family history also increases the chance of spontaneous DZ twinning, while paternal family history contributes little or nothing to this risk [2, 7]. The frequency of multiple pregnancies varies significantly among different races and ethnic groups. Women of African descent have higher rates of DZ twinning than white women, who in turn have higher rates than women of Asian descent [2]. In Japan, 1 in 250 newborns is a twin, whereas in Nigeria, 1 in 11 babies is a result of a twin gestation [2, 6]. Ovulation induction increases the occurrence of multiple pregnancies, including both dizygotic and monozygotic [4, 7].

4. Superfecundation and superfetation

Superfecundation is the fertilization of two different ova released in the same cycle, by separate acts of coitus within a short period of time. Sexual intercourse may not necessary with the same man [1, 4].

Superfetation is the fertilization of two ova released in different menstrual cycles. The implantation and development of one fetus over another fetus are theoretically possible until the uterine cavity is obliterated by 12 weeks of pregnancy. In other words, superfetation requires ovulation and fertilization during the course of an established pregnancy [1, 4].

5. Diagnosis of multiple pregnancies

5.1 Clinical evaluation

With multiple fetuses, a woman may experience excessive nausea and vomiting during the first trimester. The uterine size is typically larger than expected during the second and third trimesters.

In general, it is difficult to diagnose twins by palpation of fetal parts before the third trimester. In obese women, presence of hydramnios and overlapping fetuses are factors that make it difficult to identify twins by abdominal palpation. Palpating two or more fetal heads and or fetal poles supports a diagnosis of multiple pregnancies.

Identification of two fetal heartbeats suggests that their rates are clearly distinct from each other and from that of the mother suggests twin pregnancy.

6. Sonography

Routine prenatal ultrasound scan has proved important for early detection of multiple pregnancies. Before the advent of routine prenatal ultrasound, many twins were not diagnosed until late in gestation or delivery [2]. Separate gestational sacs with individual yolk sacs can be visualized as early as 5 weeks from the first day of the last menstrual period, and embryos with cardiac activity can usually be seen by 6 weeks by transvaginal ultrasound [2]. Prenatal sonography in multiple pregnancies is useful for the following [6]:

- Confirming a diagnosis of multiple gestations
- Determining chorionicty
- Detecting fetal anomalies
- Evaluating fetal growth
- For fetal well-being

7. Determination of chorionicity

Accurate determination of chorionicity early in pregnancy is essential to optimal obstetrics care [4]. It is a major determinant of pregnancy outcome and its determination is easiest and most reliable when assessed in the first trimester [2].

- The presence of two separate gestational sacs, each containing the fetus, and a thick dividing membrane strongly suggests dichorionic diamniotic pregnancy.
- When there is one gestational sac and a thin dividing membrane (< 2 mm) suggests monochorionic diamniotic pregnancy.
- A single gestational sac that contains two fetuses without dividing membrane suggests monochorionic monoamniotic pregnancy.

Examination of the base of the intertwin membrane is also useful for the determination of chorionicity.

- The twin peak sign appears as a triangular projection of placental tissue extending a short distance between the layers of the dividing membrane, suggesting dichorionic pregnancy.
- The T sign is the right-angle relationship between the membranes and placenta and no apparent extension of the placenta between the dividing membranes suggests monochorionic pregnancy.

The determination of chorionicity and amnionicity in the second and third trimesters can be made based on sex of fetuses, number of placentas, and thickness of the dividing membrane.

- For instance, different gender, two separate placentas, and thick dividing membrane strongly suggest dichorionic pregnancy.

After delivery, a careful visual examination of the placenta and membranes serves to establish zygosity and chorionicity in approximately two-thirds of cases [4].

8. Maternal adaptation to multiple pregnancies

The degree of maternal physiologic changes during pregnancy is exaggerated with multiple gestations. The levels of maternal hormones related to pregnancy are higher in multiple gestations than in singleton. Compared to singleton pregnancies, multiple pregnancies are associated with an increased risk of the following conditions.

- Nausea and vomiting
- Weight
- Blood volume

- Cardiac output
- Glomerular filtration rate
- Tidal volume
- Mechanical distress

9. Maternal morbidity and mortality related to multiple pregnancies

Rates of essentially every obstetrical complication are elevated with multiple pregnancies with the exception of macrosomia and post-term pregnancy. In general, these complications rise proportionally with increasing the number of fetuses.

- Hyperemesis gravidarum
- Spontaneous abortion
- Anemia
- Hypertensive disorder of pregnancy
- Abruption placentae
- Placenta previa
- Gestational diabetics
- Polyhydramnios
- Thromboembolism
- Postpartum hemorrhage
- Cesarean delivery

10. Perinatal morbidity and mortality related to multiple pregnancies

Babies who are products of multiple gestations have higher rates of:

- Low birth weight
- Preterm birth
- Malpresentation
- Premature rupture of membranes

- Umbilical cord prolapse
- Intrauterine growth restriction
- Congenital anomalies
- Neonatal and infant death and cerebral palsy

11. Fetal complications unique to multiple pregnancies

11.1 "Vanishing twin"

It refers to the loss of one member of a twin or other higher-order gestations early in pregnancy. This is typically either asymptomatic or associated with spotting or mild bleeding [2, 7]. It is responsible for lower frequency of twin or higher-order multiple gestations during the second trimester than the first trimester. For instance, if two gestational sacs are confirmed by the first-trimester ultrasound, the chance of delivering twins is 63% for women younger than 30 years and 52% for women 30 years or older [2]. Monochorionic twin gestations are at higher risk for a vanishing twin than dichorionic twins. Vanishing twin is even more common in higher-order pregnancies [2, 7]. This condition can be diagnosed with serial ultrasound with the loss of one or more fetus/fetuses.

11.2 Twin-twin transfusion syndrome (TTTS)

TTTS is exclusively a complication of monochorionic multiple pregnancies that occur in 10–15% of monochorionic diamniotic gestations [2, 5, 7]. This syndrome is characterized by unbalanced anastomoses in the placenta which leads to under perfusion of the donor twin and over perfusion of the recipient. The donor twin develops oligohydramnios and intrauterine growth restriction; the recipient experiences volume overloads which result in polyhydramnios [1–3].

TTTS can be present at any gestational age. The earlier the onset is associated with a poorer prognosis. If untreated, the mortality rates range from 80–100% [2, 7]. Both twins are at risk of demise from circulatory derangement, and the pregnancy is predisposed further for preterm delivery due to uterine overdistention with hydramnios [2].

There are three types of possible vascular anastomosis in the monochorionic placenta [1, 2, 5,]. Arteriovenous (AV), arterioarterial (AA), and venovenous (VV).

11.3 Diagnosis and staging

The two classic criteria required for antenatal diagnosis of TTTS are monochorionic diamniotic twin gestation and oligohydramnios in one amniotic sac and polyhydramnios in the other sac [1].

Once identified, TTTS is typically staged by the quintero staging system:

- Stage I- oligohydramnios, polyhydramnios sequence. Donor twin bladder is visible.

- Stage II- oligohydramnios, polyhydramnios sequence. The donor twin bladder is not visible and the doppler scan is normal.
- Stage III- oligohydramnios, polyhydramnios sequence. Donor twin bladder is not visible and doppler scans are abnormal.
- Stage IV- ascites or frank hydrops in either twin.
- Stage V- one or both fetuses have died.

When TTTS diagnosed management, it depends on gestational at diagnosis and the severity of clinical findings. There are five management options available [2]:

- Expectant management
- Septostomy
- Serial amnioreduction
- Selective termination/cord occlusion
- Fetoscopic laser photocoagulation

Generally, expectant management is not recommended in stage II or greater TTTS and selective termination is only offered in extreme cases of advanced TTTS [2].

11.4 Conjoined twins

This is a very rare event of MZ twinning resulting when the division occurs after the embryonic disc has completely formed, that is, after 13 days. It occurs with a frequency of about 1 in 50,000 pregnancies. Most conjoined twins are female, with a reported female-to-male ratio of 2:1 or 3:1 [2].

Conjoined twins are classified according to the anatomic location of the incomplete splinting [3]. The most common location is the chest (thoracopagus), followed by the anterior abdominal wall (omphalopagus), the buttocks (pygopagus), the ischium (ischiopagus), and the head (cephalopagus) [2, 3].

Conjoined twins can be diagnosed by ultrasound as early as the first trimester based on visualization of monoamnionicity and a bifid fetal pole [2].

The pregnancy termination should be offered when the diagnosis is confirmed before the age of viability. The prognosis for survival and successful separation depends on the degree of organ and vascular sharing between the two fetuses. For a better outcome, women with conjoined twins should be cared for by a multidisciplinary team [1, 2].

11.5 Intrauterine death of one fetus

Intrauterine death of one fetus in a multiple gestation can occur at any gestation. This condition is more common during the first trimester and has no or little effect on the prognosis of the surviving fetus or fetuses. After the death of one twin in a monochorionic gestation, approximately 15% of the remaining fetus also dies, while approximately 3% of remaining fetus dies in a dichorionic gestation [2].

The risk for significant neurologic morbidity is increased after intrauterine death of one fetus in a monochorioic, but not in a dichorionic gestation. The surviving twin runs the risk of cerebral palsy, microcephaly, renal cortical necrosis, and disseminated intravascular coagulation. The DIC is due to thromboplastin liberated from the dead twin that crosses via placental anastomosis to the living twin. In such cases, the maternal coagulation profile should be followed once a week to identify possible coagulation abnormalities. The dead fetus is reabsorbed if the death occurs prior to 12 weeks gestation, while the fetus shrinks and becomes dehydrated beyond this time [1, 2].

11.6 Twin reversed arterial perfusion (TRAP)

The TRAP sequence is also known as acardiac twinning and occurs only in monochorionic pregnancies. It is characterized by an acardiac-perfused twin having blood supply from a normal cotwin via arterio-arterial or vein-to-vein connection. In majority, the cotwin dies due to high output failure. The arterial pressure of the donor twin is high, the recipient twin receives the used blood from the donor. The perfused twin is often chromosomally abnormal and an extremely malformed fetus with either no heart at all or only rudimentary cardiac tissue [1, 2].

The management of TRAP is controversial. The options for management are [2, 4]:

- Expectant management
- Delivery
- Occlusion of the acardiac twin's umbilical cord by bipolar cord coagulation or laser ablation.

11.7 Twin anemia polycythemia sequence (TAPS)

This is a form of chronic fetofetal transfusion that is characterized by significant hemoglobin differences between donor and recipient twins without discrepancies in amniotic fluid volumes. The spontaneous form complicates from 3–5% of monochorionic pregnancies and it occurs in up to 13% of pregnancies after laser photocoagulation.

It is diagnosed antenatally by middle cerebral artery peak systolic velocity of more than 1.5 multiples of median (MoM) in the donor and less than 1.0 MoM in the recipient twin [1].

The options for management include expectant management and intrauterine transfusions both intraperitoneal and intravenous.

11.8 Complete hydatidiform mole with coexisting normal fetus

One of the fetuses is either complete or partial molar pregnancy, whereas the cotwin is normal fetus. The prevalence rates range from 1 in 22,000 to 100,000 pregnancies [1].

The diagnosis is usually made in the first half of pregnancy and using similar diagnostic modalities.

The possible complications are persistent and heavy bleeding, preeclampsia, preterm delivery, and persistent trophoblastic disease.

Optimal management is not known for this twin gestation. The possible options of management are termination at the time of diagnosis, and observation and pregnancy progression [1].

12. Antepartum management of multiple pregnancies

Gestational age at delivery and the adequacy of fetal growth are two important factors that most influence pregnancy outcomes [2].

The care provider should understand and advise on the following issues during antenatal care:

- Increased dietary supplement is needed for increased energy supply to the extent of 300 Kcal/day above that needed in a singleton pregnancy. Dietary supplementation includes both macronutrients and micronutrients [4].

- Increased rest at home and early cessation of work.

- Interval of antenatal contact should be more frequent.

- Multiple gestations are an increased risk for uteroplacental insufficiency. So, fetal surveillance is mandatory. It should be started at 28 weeks for triplets and higher-order pregnancies, while at 32 and 34 weeks for monochorionic twins and dichorionic twins, respectively [1, 2, 4]. The non-stress test and biophysical profile can be used and the interpretation is similar to singleton pregnancy.

- Fetal growth is monitored by ultrasound every 4 to 6 weeks beginning at 24 weeks. Twins grow at the same rate as singletons until 30 to 32 weeks gestation, after which their growth velocity slows compared with singletons. Institute of Medicine recommends women with twins and normal body mass index gain a total of 37–54 lb. weight during the pregnancy [2].

- Assess the risk for preterm birth using a transvaginal cervical length of 20 mm or less between 20- and 24-weeks' gestation and fetal fibronectin sampling [2].

- Routine use of tocolytic agents to prevent preterm delivery has no significant benefit. However, short-term use of these agents for acute tocolysis in preterm labor is helpful to gain time for administration of corticosteroids and allow transport to a tertiary care facility. Tocolytic use in multiple gestations needs careful monitoring of maternal condition as these women are at higher risk for cardiovascular complications due to exaggerated maternal cardiovascular adaptations [1, 2].

- As the numbers of fetuses increases, the prognosis of multiple pregnancies gets poorer. Now a day, there is a practice of selective fetal reduction to improve the outcome of the remaining fetus or fetuses.

13. Timing of delivery in multiple pregnancies

The timing of delivery depends on maternal and fetal complications. The available data suggest that nadir perinatal complications occur at earlier gestational ages in multiple gestations compared with singletons [2]. There is an increased risk in twin pregnancies that extend past 38 to 39 weeks gestation. Allowing a dichorionic twin gestation to go beyond 38 weeks requires convincing evidence of normal fetal growth, reassuring fetal condition as well as a woman's desire to extend the pregnancy. It is not advisable to prolong twin pregnancy past 39 weeks because of clear risk without any known benefit.

The ACOG, NICHD, and SMFM recommend the delivery of uncomplicated dichorionic twins at 38 weeks and uncomplicated monochorionic twins between 34 and 37 weeks [2].

Based on experts' opinions, it is reasonable to offer delivery of uncomplicated triples anytime between 35 and 36 weeks.

14. Mode of delivery in multiple pregnancies

Mode of delivery for patients with multiple gestations depends on the gestational age, estimated weight of the fetuses, number of fetuses, presentation of fetuses, presence or absence of complications, etc.

I. Mode of delivery in diamniotic twins

- Both twins are vertex presentation, vaginal delivery in the absence of obstetric indications for cesarean delivery.
- Twin A vertex and twin B non-vertex presentation, vaginal delivery is possible if the estimated fetal weight is 1500 g–3500 g
- Twin A non-vertex cesarean delivery is indicated.

II. Monoamniotic twins–cesarean delivery

III. Triplet and higher-order gestation–cesarean delivery

15. Intrapartum management of twin vaginal delivery

Twin pregnancy is considered high risk and needs careful preparation and multidisciplinary cooperation among obstetrics, anesthesia, nursing, and neonatology.

Both fetuses should be monitored continuously. Use of analgesic drugs is to be limited as the babies are small and rapid delivery may occur. The third stage of labor should be managed actively as these women are at high risk for postpartum hemorrhage.

Abbreviations

ACOG	American College of Obstetricians and Gynecologist
DIC	Disseminated intravascular coagulation
DZ	Dizygotic
MZ	Monozygotic

MoM	Multiples of the median
NICHD	The national institute of child health and human development
SMFM	Society for maternal-fetal medicine
TAPS	Twin anemia polycythemia sequence
TTTS	Twin-twin transfusion syndrome
TRAP	Twin reversed arterial perfusion

Author details

Mandefro Yilma Asfaw
Hawassa University, Ethiopia

*Address all correspondence to: ymande23@gmail.com

References

[1] Cunningham, Leveno, Bloom, Dashe, Hoffman, Casey, Sheffield. Multifetal Pregnancy. In: Cunningham FG, Leveno KJ, Bloom SL, Spong CY, Dashe JS, Hoffman BL, Casey BM, Sheffield JS, editors. Williams Obstetrics. 24th ed. 2014. pp. 891-920

[2] Newman RB and Unal ER. Multiple gestations. In: Gabbe, Niebly, Simpson, Landon, Galan, Jauniaux, Driscoll, Berghella, Grobman, editors. Obstetrics Normal And Problem Pregnancies. 7th ed. 2017. pp. 706-733

[3] Moore TR. Multifetal gestation and malpresentation. In: Hacker, Moore, Gambone, editors. Essentials of Obstetrics and Gynecology. 4th ed. 2007. pp. 183-188

[4] Dutta DC. Multiple pregnancy, amniotic fluid disorders, abnormalities of placenta and cord. In: Konar H, editors. DC Dutta's Textbook of Obstetrics including Perinatology and Contraception. 8th ed. 2015. pp. 233-245

[5] Bush MC and Pernoll ML. Multiple gestation. In: Dechrney AH, Nathan L, Laufer N and Roman AS, editors. Current Diagnosis and Treatment –Obstetrics and Gynecology. 11th ed. 2013. pp. 301-309

[6] Benirschke K. Multiple gestation: The biology of twinning. In: Creasy RK, Resnik R, Iams JD, Lockwood CJ, Moore TR, Greene MF, editors. Creasy and Resnik's Maternal-Fetal Medicine. 7th ed. 2014. pp. 53-65

[7] Newman RB and Rittenberg C. Multiple gestation. In: Gibbs RS, Karlan BY, Haney AF, Nygaard IE, editors. Danforth's Obstetrics and Gynecology. 10th ed. 2008. pp. 221-244

Section 2

Rare Diagnosis of Multiple Pregnancy

Chapter 5

Selective Intrauterine Growth Restriction in Monochorionic Twins

Ramya Santhanam, Anandharama Subramani Padmanabhan and Navya Nanjundegowda

Abstract

EFW of small fetus less than 10th centile/EFW discordancy >25% pathophysiology-unequal placental sharing role of vascular anastamosis in natural history-larger interfetal blood flow—type 3 better outcome than type 2 classification-based on umbilical artery doppler into three types complications—IUD of snall fetus with acute TTTS-neurological sequelae in normal twin suerviellance and management of types type 1-expectant management, close followup(weekly/biweekly doppler surviellance) and delivery by 34–35 weeks type 2-long latency to deterioration than singleton. Doppler (Ductus venosus) follow up alternate days (if abnormal DV)Or weekly (normal DV) delivery by 30–32 weeks type 3-intermittent doppler changes due to large AA anastamosis. Weekly followup if DV normal or closer follow up if abnormal. Deliver at 32 weeks role of fetal intervention-GA <24 weeks with AREDF/DV PI >95/discordancy >35%.

Keywords: siugr, monochorionic complications, fetal growth discordance, types of siugr

1. Introduction

Chorionicity decides the surveillance frequency and management in twin pregnancies than zygosity. Chorionicity is best assessed by ultrasound examination of number of placental masses, intertwin membrane thickness, examining the site of intertwin membrane attachment to placenta in cases of single fused placenta in the late first trimester or early second trimester [1].

Monochorionic twins have a higher frequency of fetal and neonatal mortality, as well as morbidities compared to dichorionic twins. Increased perinatal morbidity and mortality in monochorionic pregnancy is due to shared placenta and interplacental vascular anastomosis [2, 3].

Chronic unbalanced vascular transfusion results in twin-twin transfusion syndrome (TTTS) and twin anaemia polycythemia sequence (TAPS). Discordant placental territory results in selective intrauterine growth restriction. Unidirectional acute transfusion happens as a sequelae of single fetal demise.

Selective intrauterine fetal growth restriction (sIUGR) is a common complication in Monochorionic pregnancy. Selective fetal growth restriction is associated with increased risk of intrauterine fetal demise, prematurity and neurological adverse outcomes for one or both twins [4–8].

2. Definition and prevalence of sIUGR

The term 'selective intrauterine growth restriction' is applicable to cases meeting the following criteria.

1. Monochorionic pregnancy.

2. Estimated fetal weight (EFW) of the small fetus falls below the 10th percentile [4, 5].

3. Significant fetal weight discordance is an important element of the clinical picture. This is defined by different authors as discordance between the EFWof two foetuses>25% [9, 10]. Estimated fetal weight discordance is calculated with the following formula: (weight of the larger twin−weight of the smaller twin) × 100/weight of the larger twin.

The clinical significance of cases when both twins' EFW falls below the 10th percentile without discordance, or cases when discordance exists but the smaller fetus' EFW is above the 10th percentile, remains to be defined.

The prevalence of sIUGR ranges from 10 to 15% in monochorionic pregnancies [5, 11–13].

3. Pathophysiology of sIUGR

The principle cause for the development of sIUGR in MC twins is inadequate placental sharing [14–17] the discordance increases with increase in the discordance of placental territories between twins.

A second factor largely influencing fetal weight discordance and sIUGR in MC twins is the presence of placental vascular anastomoses/shared circulation in the monochorionic placenta [17–19].

There are basically three types of vascular anastomosis in the placenta: 1) Arterio-venous (AV) anastomoses which is characterised by unidirectional flow where a placental cotyledon is perfused by an artery from one fetus and drained by a vein going to the other fetus. This is a deep anastomosis. 2) Arterio-arterial (AA) and 3) Veno-venous (VV) anastomoses are superficially located in placenta characterised by bidirectional flow of blood; these bidirectional anastomosis have an important role in compensating the volume/pressure imbalances between foetuses.

Because of this unique vascular anastomosis in placenta and feto-fetal blood interchange via the anastamotic channels have a protective effect on the IUGR fetus, which receives blood with a normal oxygen and nutrient content from its co-twin and this is responsible for long latency before deterioration in monochorionic twins as compared to singleton.

Thus inter-twin anastomotic area, net AV transfusion and the diameter of AA anastomoses have been shown to correlate with the degree of inter-twin placental discordance. And this unique vascular anastomosis and inter fetal blood interchange is responsible for the discrepancy observed between the placental discordance and the clinical outcome.

For twins with similar placental area discordance (due to unequal sharing), twins with larger interfetal blood flow interchange (large AA anastomosis) have milder degree of clinical expression of growth restriction and better ioutcome than twins with few or smaller AA anastomosis.

Large AA anastomosis also associated with unpredictable outcomes like Double fetal demise/neurological sequelae in one or both foetuses in the absence of single fetal in type 3 IUGR.

4. Clinical implications of sIUGR

Selective IUGR is a severe complication, particularly if presenting during the second trimester, with potentially significant risks of intrauterine demise or neurological adverse outcome for both the affected IUGR and the normally grown twin [4–11].

Unique complication in monochorionic twins with sIUGR is single fetal demise/intrauterine death of growth restricted twin. And this event is associated with risk of acute feto fetal transfusion (Acute TTTS) from the normally grown twin to dead fetus due to sudden change in pressure between foetuses subsequent to single fetal demise. Acute feto-fetal transfusion is associated with 20–30% chance of neurological sequelae in surviving twin due to ischemia and hypoxia to the brain and 15–20% chance of death of larger twin due to sudden hypovolemia [20, 21].

In the absence of single fetal demise, sIUGR is associated with risk to normally grown and growth restricted twin due to following reasons:

1. To avoid the complication of single fetal demise of growth restricted twin Iatrogenic prematurity exposes the normally growing twin to face the complication associated with prematurity [22, 23].

2. In cases of type 3 sIUGR there is high risk of acute feto-fetal transfusion accidents in utero due to the large AA anastomosis in the placenta and this event increases the risk of neurological complications in both the foetuses [4, 7, 24].

5. Screening for sIUGR in monochorionic pregnancy

Do not use abdominal palpation or symphysis-fundal height measurements to monitor for fetal growth restriction in women with a monochorionic twin [25].

Ultrasonography is the screening modality of choice. At each ultrasound scan from 16 weeks, assesss fetal biometry and calculate the fetal weight discordance in addition to amniotic fluid level assessment. Surveillance to be conducted every 2 weeks [25].

On surveillance if there is an EFW discordance of 25% or more between twins and the EFW of any of the babies is below the 10th centile for gestational age the women should be referred to a tertiary level fetal medicine centre [25].

6. Classification of sIUGR

In singleton and Dichorionic twin pregnancies, doppler waveform of umbilical artery is commonly used to diagnose, plan surveillance frequency for fetus with growth restriction due to uteroplacental insufficiency [26].

In monochorionic pregnancies the changes in umbilical artery waveform represents combined effect of uteroplacental insufficiency and inter-twin vascular anastamosis [22, 27–31].

Based on the characteristics of diastolic flow of umbilical artery Doppler waveform selective fetal growth restriction in monochorionic twin pregnancies is categorised into following three types:

1. Type I sIUGR characterised by presence of diastolic flow in umbilical artery waveform.

2. Type II sIUGR characterised by persistent absence/reversal of flow in umbilical artery Doppler waveform.

3. Type III sIUGR characterised by intermittent absence/reversal of flow in umbilical artery Doppler waveform (iAREDF) [22, 27, 28]. These types not only correlate with distinct clinical forms but also with distinct patterns of placental anastomoses

Type 3 also been defined as cyclical pattern because of intermittent changes in Doppler waveform. This intermittent changes happens because of the presence of large interplacental AA anastomosis causing waveforms pattern due to transmission of blood from larger to smaller twin [22, 27].

To diagnose type 3 sIUGR sweep speed of Doppler to be kept low and longer traces has to be observed.

Doppler changes in selective fetal growth restriction are evident early in pregnancy and there is a long latency between onset of Doppler changes and progression because of the presence of shared vascular anastomosis. The clinical outcomes are considered; good in type 1 cases, increased risk of deterioration observed in type 2 cases with poor prognosis. Type 3 sIUGR have comparatively better prognosis than type 2 cases due to large AA anastomosis. Large AA anastomosis also increases the risk of antepartum brain hypoxic and ischemic injury to both the twins with a unpredictable outcome in type 3 cases [4, 24].

7. Differential diagnosis

Monochorionic pregnancies need fortnightly surviellance to rule out evolving complications [21]. during followup ultrasound fetal biometry, estimated fetal weight, single vertical pocket measurement made and weight difference calculated at each visit. Detailed anatomical evaluation with extended cardiac evaluation done around 20–22 weeks in both twins. Doppler assessment of umbilical artery, middle cerebral artery done in each visit.

Detailed evaluation rules out the common differential diagnosis of SIUGR which is TTTS characterised by EFW discordance with a characteristic liquor discordance between twins (SVP <2 cm in donor and SVP >10 cm in recipient) [21].

8. Type I sIUGR

8.1 Definition and placental features

Type I sIUGR is characterised by presence of diastolic flow in umbilical artery of smaller twin (**Figure 1**). In twin pregnancy with unequal placental sharing there should be a linear relation between shared placental territory and the fetal weight difference between twins. In selective fetal growth restriction this ratio is lower that is the actual fetal weight discordance between twins is lower compared to the placental territory discordance. This is because of the shared vascular anastomosis favours the blood flow from larger to smaller twin in a compensatory manner attenuating the effects of unequal placental territory sharing (placental insufficiency of smaller twin) [7, 16, 17].

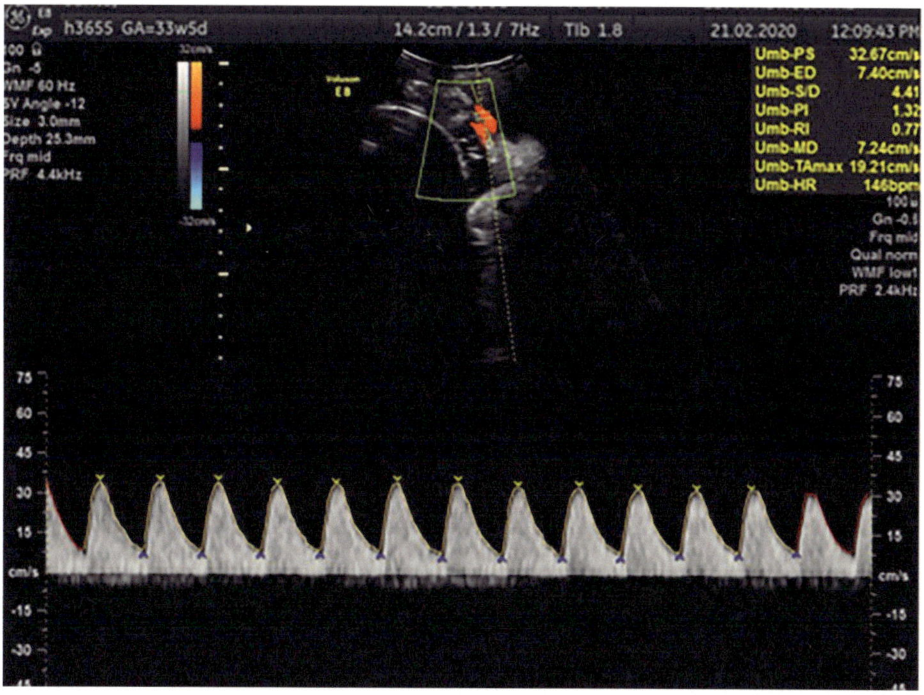

Figure 1.
PD of umbilical artery—End diastolic flow noted in smaller twin (type I).

8.2 Clinical evolution and suggested management

Type I cases are generally associated with good outcomes and 90–95% perinatal survival. Intrauterine fetal death rates in type I sIUGR is around 2–4% [7, 24, 30]. and neurological damage was reported in less than 5% of cases [3, 25].

The deterioration or worsening of Doppler parameters in smaller twin is slower than the singleton growth restricted fetus. Most cases of type I sIUGR will remain without progression till delivery.

Smaller twin of sIUGR type I usually will show a linear growth curve without deterioration. Type I sIUGR cases need expectant management with close follow-up to rule out progression to type II. Type I cases need weekly ultrasound and Doppler surveillance.

Elective delivery planned around 34–36 weeks in type I sIUGR cases without deterioration [21].

9. Type II sIUGR

9.1 Definition and placental features

Type II sIUGR pattern is characterised by persistently absent or reversed end-diastolic flow in the umbilical artery (**Figure 2**). Type II sIUGR cases have more severe placental discordance than type I cases [16]. Despite severe placental territory discordance the fetal weight difference between twins is lower illustrating the attenuating effect of shared vascular anastomosis between twins [16].

Type II sIUGR have smaller diameter of placental vascular anastomosis and fewer anastomosis than type I sIUGR cases. Hence the protective effect of vascular anastomosis is less efficient in type II sIUGR cases.

Thus, placental insufficiency in type II is far more severe than in type I and cannot be fully compensated by inter-twin transfusion.

Fetal deterioration defined by abnormal progression of Doppler wave forms in ductus venosus happen before 30 weeks of gestation in 70–90% cases of type II sIUGR [4, 7, 22, 24].

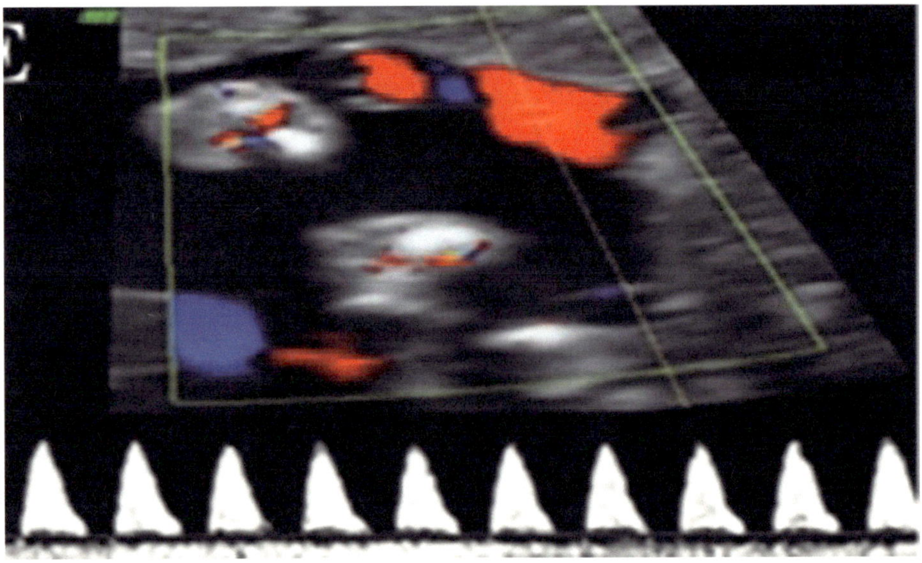

Figure 2.
PD of umbilical artery—Absent end diastolic flow in smaller twin (type II sIUGR).

9.2 Clinical evolution

Because of the protective effect of shared vascular anastomosis there is a longer latency period between onset of absent or reversed end diastolic flow in umbilical artery to ductus venosus Doppler decompensation (Pulsatality index >95th centile/'a' wave absence or reversal) or pathologically abnormal biophysical profile warranting delivery in monochorionic twins (approximately 10 weeks) compared to singleton pregnancy with similar Doppler findings (3–4 weeks) [7, 22].

At the same time the gestational age of onset of abnormal Doppler finding (A/REDF) is much earlier in complicated monochorionic twins (20 weeks) compared to singletons (27 weeks) with clinical deterioration warranting iatrogenic premature delivery around 30 weeks in 90% cases [7, 22].

Elective delivery is indicated in most of these pregnancies earlier than 30 weeks of gestation [7, 22] with only a small minority surviving in utero beyond 32 weeks. Incidence of single fetal demise of smaller twin in type II sIUGR is around 20–30% [3].

9.3 Management

Close fetal surveillance with Doppler evaluation of umbilical and ductus venosus Doppler is practiced although type II sIUGR complicated twins have a longer latency period before clinical deterioration.

Ductus venosus Doppler is useful tool to plan timing of delivery in type II sIUGR cases as DV Doppler abnormality is the predictor of imminent fetal death. Weekly follow up is ideal if ductus venosus Doppler is normal and more frequent follow up scheduled if ductus venosus shows abnormality (pulsatility index >95th centile/absent or reversal of a wave of DV Doppler). Biophysical profile can be included as surveillance tool after fetal viability is reached.

Elective delivery is indicated in most of these pregnancies earlier than 30 weeks of gestation [7, 22] with only a small minority surviving in utero beyond 32 weeks.

9.4 Role of fetal intervention

Fetal therapy is preformed in:

1. severe cases diagnosed before 24 weeks of gestation (cases with severe discordance >35% before viability or ductus venosus Doppler pulsatility index >95th centile before 24 weeks).

2. if smaller fetus shows signs of imminent fetal death (ductus venosus Doppler showing absent or reversal of a wave) before fetal viability (before 24 weeks of gestation).

Fetal intervention methods:

1. Cord occlusion—Bipolar cord coagulation of smaller fetus [32–34]. Studies showed 90% survival rate in normal fetus after procedure [33]. Cord occlusion is the preferred fetal intervention in indicated cases of sIUGR.

2. fetoscopic laser coagulation of intertwin anastomoses [32, 34] studies found remarkable mortality rates in normally grown fetus (20–30%) with laser coagulation [35]. Fetoscopic laser coagulation of vascular anastomosis associated with increased risk of preterm labour, double fetal demise. Laser coagulation is technically difficult in sIUGR cases than twin to twin transfusion cases due to absence of placental flattening (no polyhydramnios in sIUGR) and presence

of amniotic fluid in smaller twin sac hampering the visualisation of vascular equator [32] all yjese are associated with increased complication rates with laser surgery.

10. Type III sIUGR

10.1 Characteristic doppler findings and placental features

Type III sIUGR is defined by the intermittent Absent/Reversed End Diastolic Flow in the Umbilical artery Doppler of the growth restricted twin. This alternation in positive waveform and absent/reversal of diastolic flow in umbilical artery is characteristic of Monochorionic twin due to presence of shared vascular anastomosis in the placenta (**Figure 3**). This unique wave pattern indicates the presence of a large placental Arterio-Arterial anastomosis [29, 32], facilitating transmission of the systolic waveforms of one twin into the umbilical cord of the other twin.

This Doppler pattern of intermittent absent/reversal of flow in end diastolic flow of umbilical artery can also be observed in rare cases of uncomplicated monochorionic pregnancies with very close cord insertions and even in pregnancies complicated with TTTS [31].

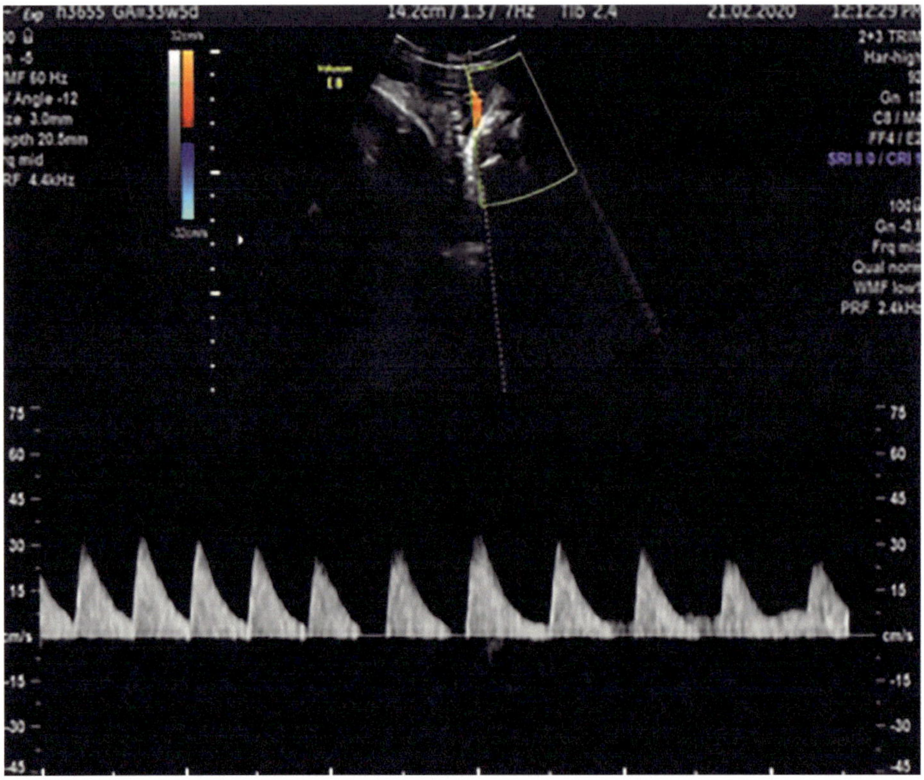

Figure 3.
PD of umbilical artery—intermittent absent end diastolic flow—Type III SIUGR.

10.2 Clinical evolution and pathophysiological basis

The sign is often more pronounced near the placental cord insertion site. Maternal breathing to be withheld during Doppler assessment to avoid artefacts associated with maternal movements. A low sweep speed pulse Doppler setting is ideal to identify the cyclic changes, otherwise it can easily be missed and may lead to under-diagnosis of type III sIUGR cases.

Placental territory discordance is highest in type III sIUGR cases [16]. Large Arterio-arterial anastomosis compensates the imbalance because of the massive transfusion from larger to smaller twin. This large Arterio-arterial anastomosis increases risk of acute feto-fetal transfusion episodes in the event of transient bradycardia of the smaller twin, increasing the risk of unexpected intrauterine death of the growth restricted fetus and ischemic brain injury in the normally grown twin [16].

Normally grown fetus is at risk of hypertrophic cardiomyopathy-like changes (20% cases) as it has to supply blood for smaller twin through large AA anastomosis [36]. So in a way larger twin works as pump twin (in cases of monochorionic pregnancy with acardiac fetus) and experiences cardiac strain. Such cardiac changes are not associated with a immediate poorer neonatal prognosis [37], although the long-term impact on cardiac function has not been evaluated.

IUGR type III pregnancies are characterised by an apparently benign evolution due to the compensating effect of the large Arterio-arterial allowing survival of the severe growth restricted fetus beyond 32 or 34 weeks without any sign of hypoxic deterioration.

Presence of large arterio-arterial anastomosis is associated with risk of fetal demise of smaller twin in 15–20% cases with a risk of hypoxic brain damage in normally grown twin due to acute feto-fetal transfusion in 15–30% cases [4, 26].

However, type III sIUGR is associated with a risk of unpredictable fetal demise of the growth restricted fetus in up to 15–20% of cases. There is also risk of brain damage of the normally grown fetus, even when both foetuses are born alive, affecting as many as 15–30% of cases [4, 24]. These complications are due to acute feto-fetal hemorrhagic accidents through the large Arterio-Arterial anastomosis happening during transient bradycardic episodes of the smaller twin.

10.3 Clinical management of type III sIUGR pregnancies

Management of type III sIUGR represents a challenge.

Prognosis is better than type II cases due to protective effect of smaller twin by the arterio-arterial anastomosis. Same anastomosis is associated with increased risk of unpredictable adverse outcomes like single fetal demise, double fetal demise, hypoxic and ischemic damage to normally grown twin and its sequelae.

Risk associated with type III sIUGR cases are due large Arterio-arterial anastamosis, a high inter fetal weight discordance, and a short distance between the cord insertions.

Weekly ultrasound and Doppler surveillance if ductus venosus doppler is normal and closer followup if ductus venosus flow becomes abnormal.

Elective delivery around 32-34 weeks of gestation [21], to reduce the opportunity for unexpected adverse outcomes.

10.4 Role of fetal intervention

Fetal therapy is considered for very early (before fetal viability)severe cases,cases with extreme estimated fetal weight discordance(>35% discordance).

Cord occlusion is preferred method of fetal intervention. Laser coagulation is also feasible in type III pregnancies, but it is associated with more technical difficulties than in type II [35].

11. Flow chart of management

See **Figure 4**.

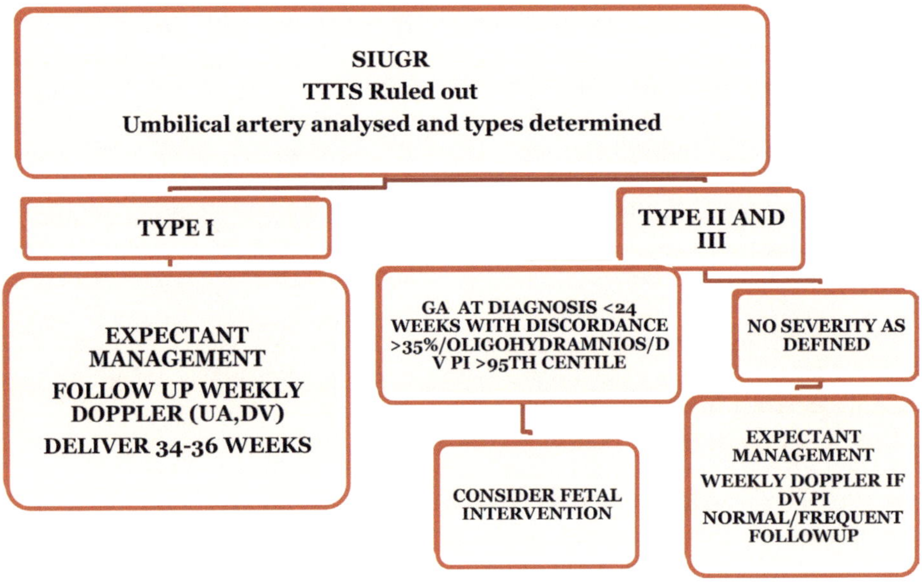

Figure 4.
Flow chart of management of selective fetal growth restriction.

Author details

Ramya Santhanam[1*], Anandharama Subramani Padmanabhan[2]
and Navya Nanjundegowda[3]

1 Consultant Fetomaternal Medicine, Gynaecology and Genetics, Narbhavi Hospital, Kanchipuram, Tamilnadu, India

2 Radiologist, Head quarter Government Hospital, Kanchipuram, Tamilnadu, India

3 Consultant Fetal Medicine and Genetics, Rainbow Children's Hospital, Bengaluru, Karnataka, India

*Address all correspondence to: sramya.medico@gmail.com

References

[1] Glinianaia SV, Obeysekera MA, Sturgiss S, Bell R. Stillbirth and neonatal mortality in monochorionic and dichorionic twins: A population-based study. Human Reproduction. 2011;**26**:2549-2557. (Level II-3)

[2] Kilby MD. Bricker L on behalf of the Royal College of Obstetricians and Gynaecologists. Management of monochorionic twin pregnancy. BJOG. 2016;**124**:e1-e45

[3] Geipel A, Berg C, Katalinic A, Plath H, Hansmann M, Germer U, et al. Prenatal diagnosis and obstetric outcomes in triplet pregnancies in relation to chorionicity. BJOG. 2005;**112**:554-558. (Level II-3)

[4] Gratacós E, Carreras E, Becker J, et al. Prevalence of neurological damage in monochorionic twins with selective intrauterine growth restriction and intermittent absent or reversed end-diastolic umbilical artery flow. Ultrasound in Obstetrics & Gynecology. 2004;**24**:159e63

[5] Sebire NJ, Snijders RJ, Hughes K, et al. The hidden mortality of monochorionic twin pregnancies. British Journal of Obstetrics and Gynaecology. 1997;**104**:1203e7

[6] Victoria A, Mora G, Arias F. Perinatal outcome, placental pathology, and severity of discordance in monochorionic and dichorionic twins. Obstetrics and Gynecology. 2001;**97**:310e5

[7] Gratacós E, Lewi L, Munoz B, et al. A classification system for selective intrauterine growth restriction in monochorionic pregnancies according to umbilical artery Doppler flow in the smaller twin. Ultrasound in Obstetrics & Gynecology. 2007;**30**:28e34

[8] Lewi L, Gucciardo L, Huber A, et al. Clinical outcome and placental characteristics of monochorionic diamniotic twin pairs with early- and late-onset discordant growth. American Journal of Obstetrics and Gynecology. 2008;**199**:511.e1e7

[9] O'Brien WF, Knuppel RA, Scerbo JC, Rattan PK. Birth weight in twins: An analysis of discordancy and growth retardation. Obstetrics and Gynecology. 1986;**67**:483e6

[10] Erkkola R, Ala-Mello S, Piiroinen O, Kero P, Sillanpää M. Growth discordancy in twin pregnancies: A risk factor not detected by measurements of biparietal diameter. Obstetrics and Gynecology. 1985;**66**:203e6

[11] Ortibus E, Lopriore E, Deprest J, et al. The pregnancy and long-term neurodevelopmental outcome of monochorionic diamniotic twin gestations: A multicenter prospective cohort study from the first trimester onward. American Journal of Obstetrics and Gynecology. 2009;**200**:494.e1e8

[12] Lewi L, Van Schoubroeck D, Gratacós E, et al. Monochorionic diamniotic twins: Complications and management options. Current Opinion in Obstetrics & Gynecology. 2003;**15**:177e94

[13] Acosta-Rojas R, Becker J, Munoz-Abellana B, et al. Twin chorionicity and the risk of adverse perinatal outcome. International Journal of Gynaecology and Obstetrics. 2007;**96**:98e102

[14] Chang YL, Chang SD, Chao AS, Hsieh PC, Wang CN, Wang TH. Clinical outcome and placental territory ratio of monochorionic twin pregnancies and

selective intrauterine growth restriction with different types of umbilical artery Doppler. Prenatal Diagnosis. 2009;**29**:253e6

[15] Fick AL, Feldstein VA, Norton ME, et al. Unequal placental sharing and birth weight discordance in monochorionic diamniotic twins. American Journal of Obstetrics and Gynecology. 2006;**195**:178e83

[16] Lewi L, Cannie M, Blickstein I, et al. Placental sharing, birthweight discordance, and vascular anastomoses in monochorionic diamniotic twin placentas. American Journal of Obstetrics and Gynecology. 2007;**197**:587.e1e8

[17] Denbow ML, Cox P, Taylor M, Hammal DM, Fisk NM. Placental angioarchitecture in monochorionic twin pregnancies: Relationship to fetal growth, fetofetal transfusion syndrome, and pregnancy outcome. American Journal of Obstetrics and Gynecology. 2000;**182**:417e26

[18] Machin GA. Velamentous cord insertion in monochorionic twin gestation. An added risk factor. The Journal of Reproductive Medicine. 1997;**42**:785e9

[19] Hack KE, Nikkels PG, Koopman-Esseboom C, et al. Placental characteristics of monochorionic diamniotic twin pregnancies in relation to perinatal outcome. Placenta. 2008;**29**:976e81

[20] Bejar R, Vigliocco G, Gramajo H, et al. Antenatal origin of neurologic damage in newborn infants. II. Multiple gestations. American Journal of Obstetrics and Gynecology. 1990;**162**:1230e6

[21] Khalil A, Rodgers M, Baschat A, Bhide A, Gratacos E, Hecher K, et al ISUOG Practice Guidelines: role of ultrasound in twin pregnancy. Ultrasound Obstet Gynecol. Feb 2016;**47**(2):247-63. DOI: 10.1002/uog.15821. Erratum in: Ultrasound Obstet Gynecol. Jul 2018;**52**(1):140. PMID: 26577371

[22] Vanderheyden TM, Fichera A, Pasquini L, et al. Increased latency of absent enddiastolic flow in the umbilical artery of monochorionic twin fetuses. Ultrasound in Obstetrics & Gynecology. 2005;**26**:44e9

[23] Gratacós E, Lewi L, Carreras E, et al. Incidence and characteristics of umbilical artery intermittent absent and/or reversed end-diastolic flow in complicated and uncomplicated monochorionic twin pregnancies. Ultrasound in Obstetrics & Gynecology. 2004;**23**:456e60

[24] Ishii K, Murakoshi T, Takahashi Y, et al. Perinatal outcome of monochorionic twins with selective intrauterine growth restriction and different types of umbilical artery doppler under expectant management. Fetal Diagnosis and Therapy. 2009;**26**:157e61

[25] Gibson JL, Castleman JS, Meher S, Kilby MD. Updated guidance for the management of twin and triplet pregnancies from the National Institute for Health and Care Excellence guidance, UK: What's new that may improve perinatal outcomes? Acta Obstet Gynecol Scand. Feb 2020;**99**(2):147-152. DOI: 10.1111/aogs.13785. Epub 2019 Dec 23. PMID: 31799724

[26] Sebire NJ. Umbilical artery Doppler revisited: Pathophysiology of changes in intrauterine growth restriction revealed. Ultrasound in Obstetrics & Gynecology. 2003;**21**:419e22

[27] Hecher K, Jauniaux E, Campbell S, et al. Artery-to-artery anastomosis in

monochorionic twins. American Journal of Obstetrics and Gynecology. 1994;**171**:570e2

[28] Gratacós E, Van Schoubroeck D, Carreras E, et al. Impact of laser coagulation in severe twinetwin transfusion syndrome on fetal Doppler indices and venous blood flow volume. Ultrasound in Obstetrics & Gynecology. 2002;**20**:125e30

[29] Wee LY, Taylor MJ, Vanderheyden T, et al. Transmitted arterio-arterial anastomosis waveforms causing cyclically intermittent absent/reversed enddiastolic umbilical artery flow in monochorionic twins. Placenta. 2003;**24**:772e8

[30] Gaziano E, Gaziano C, Brandt D. Doppler velocimetry determined redistribution of fetal blood flow: Correlation with growth restriction in diamniotic monochorionic and dizygotic twins. American Journal of Obstetrics and Gynecology. 1998;**178**:1359e67

[31] Bajoria R, Wee LY, Anwar S, et al. Outcome of twin pregnancies complicated by single intrauterine death in relation to vascular anatomy of the monochorionic placenta. Human Reproduction. 1999;**14**:2124e30

[32] Quintero RA, Bornick PW, Morales WJ, Allen MH. Selective photocoagulation of communicating vessels in the treatment of monochorionic twins with selective growth retardation. American Journal of Obstetrics and Gynecology. 2001;**185**:689e96

[33] Parra-Cordero M, Bennasar M, Martínez JM, Eixarch E, Torres X, Gratacos E. Cord occlusion in monochorionic twins with early selective intrauterine growth restriction and abnormal umbilical artery Doppler: A consecutive series of 90 cases. Fetal Diagnosis and Therapy. 2016;**39**:186e91

[34] Lewi L, Gratacós E, Ortibus E, et al. Pregnancy and infant outcome of 80 consecutive cord coagulations in complicated monochorionic multiple pregnancies. American Journal of Obstetrics and Gynecology. 2006;**194**:782e9

[35] Valsky DV, Eixarch E, Martinez JM, Gratacos E. Selective intrauterine growth restriction in monochorionic diamniotic twin pregnancies. Prenatal Diagnosis. 2010;**30**:719e26

[36] Munoz-Abellana B, Hernandez-Andrade E, Figueroa-Diesel H, Ferrer Q, Acosta-Rojas R, Cabero L, et al. Hypertrophic cardiomyopathy-like changes in monochorionic twin pregnancies with selective intrauterine growth restriction and intermittent absent/reversed end-diastolic flow in the umbilical artery. Ultrasound in Obstetrics & Gynecology. 2007;**30**:977e82

[37] Gardiner HM, Matsui H, Roughton M, Greenwald SE, Diemert A, Taylor MJ, et al. Cardiac function in 10-year-old twins following different fetal therapies for twinetwin transfusion syndrome. Ultrasound in Obstetrics & Gynecology. 2014;**43**:652e7

Chapter 6

Recent Updates in the Management of Monochorionic Twin Pregnancy

Rafiea Jeddy

Abstract

Monochorionic pregnancies are at high risk of developing severe complications leading to high perinatal morbidity and mortality. About 15% of these twins have unidirectional anastomosis of the placenta, which is responsible for the major complications specific to monochorionic pregnancies. An important first step in the management is the identification of the chorionicity. Once it is identified, a close follow-up every 2 weeks is vital to allow early detection of complications and their management. Approximately 1 in 10 monochorionic pregnancies develops twin-to-twin transfusion syndrome, congenital anomalies, anaemia polycythaemia sequence, selective intrauterine growth restriction and intrauterine death of a co-twin. Rare complications that can occur are twin reversed arterial perfusion syndrome. Timely screening and detection of all such complications can lead to appropriate intervention such as in utero foetoscopic laser treatment. These interventions can increase the survival rate of at least one or both twins with reduced neonatal morbidity. Besides, early detection can facilitate parents to have an informed choice to decide if the prognosis of the pregnancy is otherwise not good.

Keywords: monochorionic, updates, management, twin to twin transfusion, selective growth restriction, twin anaemia polycythaemia

1. Introduction

The incidence of twin pregnancy in the United States in recent times is approximately 3% [1]. With advancing age, different ethnic populations and advanced use of assisted reproduction technology, the incidence of dizygotic twins is far more common and accounts for 70% of all twin gestations. However, the incidence of monozygotic twins remains mostly constant worldwide and accounts for 3–5 per thousand births. The incidence of monochorionic twins is 1 in 300 pregnancies. In about 15% of these twins, there is an imbalance in foetal circulation. This results in conditions like twin-to-twin transfusion syndrome (TTTS), twin anaemia polycythaemia syndrome (TAPS), twin reversed arterial perfusion syndrome (TRAP), selective intrauterine growth restriction (sIUGR) and death of a co-twin.

In this chapter, we discuss the latest updates in the management of monochorionic twin pregnancy.

2. Chronicity and twinning

The most essential component of foetal well-being in twin pregnancy is the determination of the placental chronicity. Placental physiology has a vital impact on foetal and neonatal outcomes. Monozygotic twins develop when a single sperm fertilises with a single ovum during conception. Post conception, if the splitting of the egg occurs 2–3 days post fertilisation, it results in dichorionic, diamniotic twins. Approximately 30% of monozygotic twins are diamniotic and dichorionic. A splitting of egg 3–8 days post-conception results in monochorionic and diamniotic twins. About 70% of monozygotic twins are monochorionic diamniotic. If splitting occurs 9–12 days after fertilisation, it results in monoamniotic monochorionic twins.

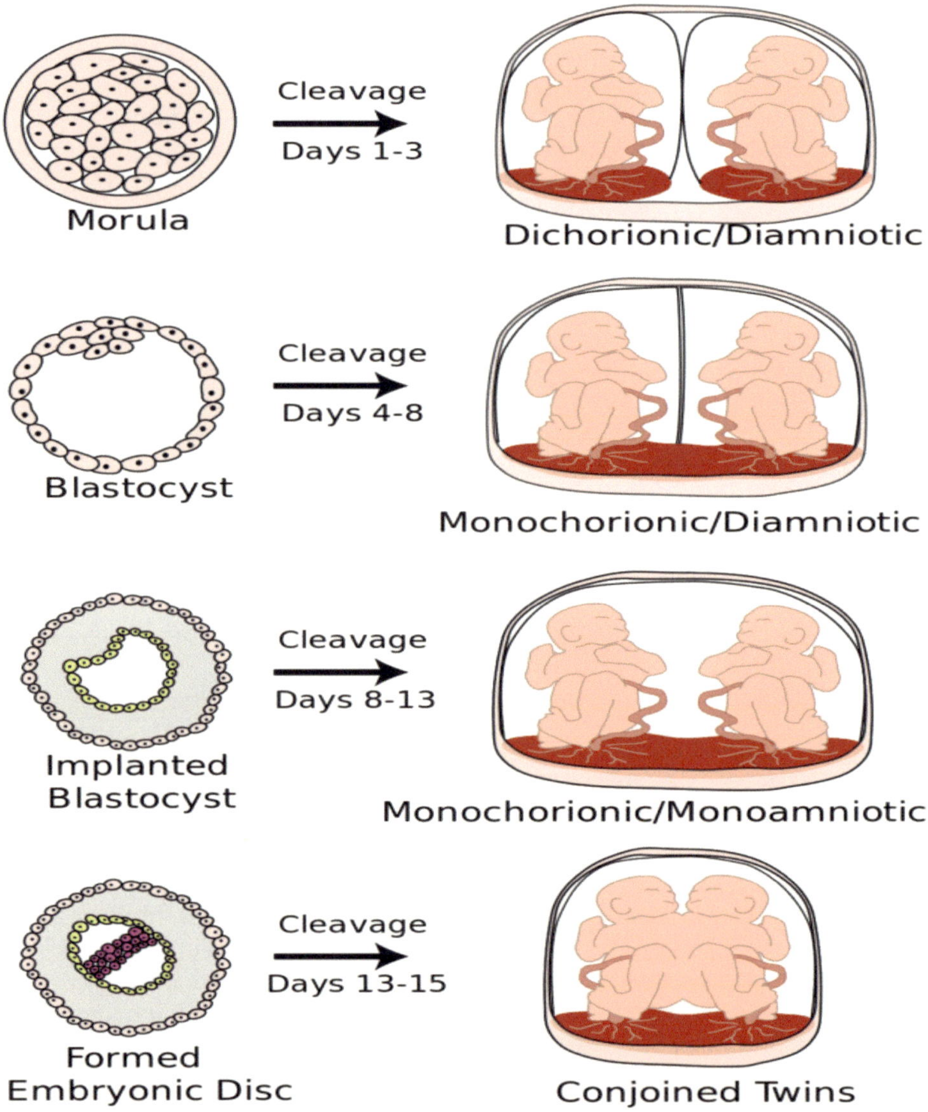

Figure 1.
Courtesy—Google images.

The incidence of these twins is only 1%. There is a well-documented increased incidence of second-trimester loss, congenital anomalies, and prematurity in these twins. A splitting after 12 days fertilisation can result in conjoined twins (**Figure 1**).

As a result of a single placenta, monochorionic twins have substantial vascular communications between the two foetal circulations. In 80% of cases, the vascular anastomosis is bidirectional, which rarely leads to a haemodynamic imbalance between foetal circulations. However, it allows a direct vascular connection between the twins with an increased risk of foetal death [2, 3].

In 15% of monochorionic pregnancies, the placenta has have a predominance of unidirectional vascular anastomosis which results in twin-to-twin transfusion syndrome (TTTS) [2]. Other morbidities exclusive to monochorionic pregnancies are:

- Intrauterine growth restriction (sIUGR)
- Twin anaemia polycythaemia sequence (TAPS)
- Neurodevelopmental morbidity
- Trap reversal arterial perfusion syndrome (TRAP)
- The death of a single twin and its effects on the second twin

3. The role of ultrasound in determining chronicity and amnionicity

It is vital that all women with twin pregnancies should be offered an ultrasound examination between 11 + 0 and 13 + 6 weeks of gestation (crown-rump length 45–84 mm [2]. This is crucial to assess foetal viability, gestational age and chronicity. In monochorionic diamniotic pregnancies, the intertwin membrane becomes progressively thin after 9 weeks. A characteristic 'T' sign is seen on ultrasound with a 100% sensitivity and greater than 98% specificity for detecting monochorionic diamniotic gestation [4]. On the other hand, in dichorionic diamniotic pregnancies, a 'twin peak' or lambda sign is characteristic with a sensitivity greater than 97% and specificity of 100% in predicting chronicity [4]. It is a good practice to determine the amnionicity at the same time and document it as well (**Figure 2**).

Other sonographic signs to determine chronicity, especially when women present after 14 weeks of gestation, include number of placental masses, number of

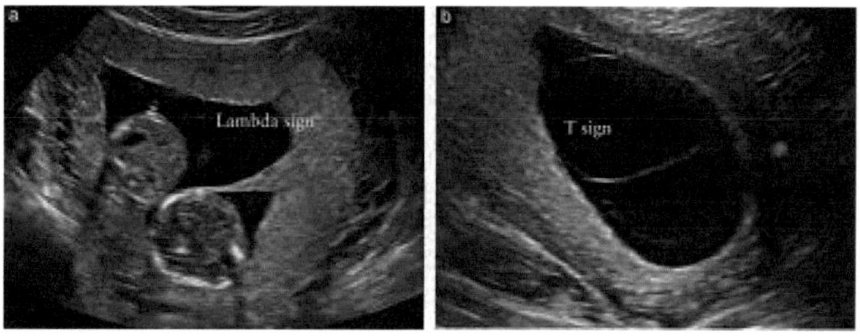

Figure 2.
Courtesy: (obgyn.onlinelibrary.wiley.com).

gestational sacs and concordant sex of the foetuses but the most valuable sign is the intertwin membrane using 2-dimensional ultrasound which is considered as highly accurate with very high sensitivity and specificity. The reliability of the number of placental masses may become arguable, as it is not unusual for dichorionic placentae to be commonly adjacent to each other and give appearance of a single mass. It is also noted that 3% of monochorionic twin pregnancies may have two placental masses on ultrasound, the presence of which does not prevent the presence of vascular anastomoses. It is likely that using a combination of ultrasound features, rather than one, would be more accurate [5].

4. The clinical implications of increased nuchal translucency in 11–13 weeks in twin pregnancy based on chronicity

Several studies have reported a comparison of increased nuchal translucency versus normal nuchal translucency in both dichorionic and monochorionic twins. However, a recent study has demonstrated that monochorionic twin pregnancies with increased nuchal translucency, but no chromosomal abnormalities had a higher incidence of structural anomalies and twin-specific complications. The most likely cause of increased nuchal translucency in these twins could be because of their unique vascular anastomoses which can lead to conditions like cardiac dysfunction, anaemia and possibly twin-to-twin transfusion syndrome. The studies indicated that detection of increased nuchal translucency is important in the early prediction of twin-specific complications although the appropriate intervention in such cases remains controversial [6]. Similarly, a discordance in nuchal translucency measurements of more than 20% is often seen in those cases of monochorionic diamniotic twin pregnancies that develop early twin to twin transfusion than those with normal outcomes [7]. The risk of TTTS and early intrauterine death in such cases is up to 30%. Such cases should be discussed with the foetal medicine expert and should be offered a detailed ultrasound and karyotyping [5].

As for the chromosomal screening, it is recommended in monochorionic twins when aneuploidy sceening is offered nuchal translucency should be used in conjunction with first-trimester serum markers (combined screening test) at 11 + 0 weeks to 13 + 6 weeks of gestation (crown–rump length 45–84 mm). Studies have shown that although non-invasive prenatal testing has a high screening efficiency in a singleton pregnancy, its performance in twin pregnancies remains unstable. Hence, it should be carefully used in the screening of chromosomal abnormalities in twins [8].

As it is well recognised that screening and diagnostic testing in twins are more complex than in singleton pregnancy, hence comprehensive counselling should be provided by health care experts before tests are taken. Health care providers should inform couples regarding the complex decisions which may be potentially required especially in cases of monochorionic twin pregnancy.

With regards to performing amniocentesis in monochorionic twins, if monochorionicity has been confirmed before 14 weeks of gestation and there is no gross discordant in growth of foetuses, it is acceptable to sample only one amniotic sac. Otherwise, both amniotic sacs need to be sampled as the rare possibility of discordant chromosomal anomalies in monochorionic pregnancy cannot be ruled out. Chorionic villus sampling (CVS) in monochorionic pregnancy will sample only the single placenta. This could miss the rare discordant chromosomal anomalies. Discordance for most of the common human aneuploidies (trisomy's 13, 18 and 21, Turner syndrome and triploidy) has been reported in monochorionic twin pairs. In the event of such a case, a selective reduction by umbilical cord occlusion can be offered from 16 weeks onwards, with a survival rate of more than 80% for the healthy twin. It is extremely important to provide detailed counselling in such complex cases to the parents by foetal medicine experts [5].

5. Dating of the twins

It is recommended that the pregnancy should be dated according to the crown-rump length of the larger twin. Dating should take place when the crown-rump length is between 45 mm and 84 mm (equivalent to 11 + 0 to 13 + 6 weeks of gestation). Twins, if seen after 14 weeks, should be dated according to the head circumference of the larger twin [9].

6. Labelling of the twins

Labelling of twins should follow a reliable and steady strategy with options according to their site; for example right or left, upper or lower or according to the insertion of cord in relation to placental membrane insertion as recorded during first trimester scans. If there is a discordance in the twins, a description such as 'potential recipient' can be used for labelling. It is important to note that twins as seen on ultrasound may not be delivered in the same sequence especially during a caesarean section. Thus, it is strongly recommended to rescan the women just before performing a caesarean especially in cases of twin congenital abnormality like cardiac defects or diaphragmatic hernia and before any surgical intervention [5].

7. The antenatal care of women with monochorionic diamniotic twin pregnancy

It is recommended that monochorionic diamniotic pregnancy should have hospital-based care. If any complications arise, then tertiary care should be advised. Women with monochorionic diamniotic twin pregnancy require a good and strong emotional support throughout the pregnancy bearing in mind the foetal morbidity and mortality associated with the twins. All efforts should be made to reduce their anxiety, and comprehensive counselling should be done at the booking visit. The screening and diagnostic tests and their complexity should also be discussed at the initial visit.

General advice regarding diet and lifestyle should be given [10]. It should be emphasised that women with twin pregnancies are more prone to anaemia, pre-eclampsia, gestational diabetes, varicose veins as well as increased risk of venous thromboembolism, antepartum and postpartum haemorrhage. All usual antenatal screening blood tests should be advised as singleton pregnancy. If anaemia is detected, iron should be commenced in early pregnancy along with folic acid. Vitamin D should also be started from early pregnancy if a woman is deficient in vitamin D.

A prophylaxis dose of Aspirin 100–150 mg is recommended from 12 weeks to 36 weeks of pregnancy if other risk factors are present such as:

Previous history of hypertensive disorders in pregnancy; chronic hypertension in pregnancy; chronic kidney disease; history of Type 1 or type 2 diabetes; primigravida; history of autoimmune conditions such as antiphospholipid syndrome or systemic lupus erythematosus; age greater than 40 years; family history of pre-eclampsia or obesity greater than 35 at first visit [10].

The antenatal and ultrasound visit schedule for monochorionic diamniotic twins (**Figure 3**).

Most recent studies suggest a structured ultrasound schedule for the antenatal management of monochorionic twin pregnancy. It is now generally accepted that after the first visit and ultrasound at 12 weeks, monochorionic pregnancies should have antenatal visits every 2 weeks from 16 weeks onwards. At every visit, an ultrasound should be performed for the early detection of twin transfusion syndrome and twin anaemia polycythaemia syndrome, as early detection of these conditions results in a better perinatal outcome.

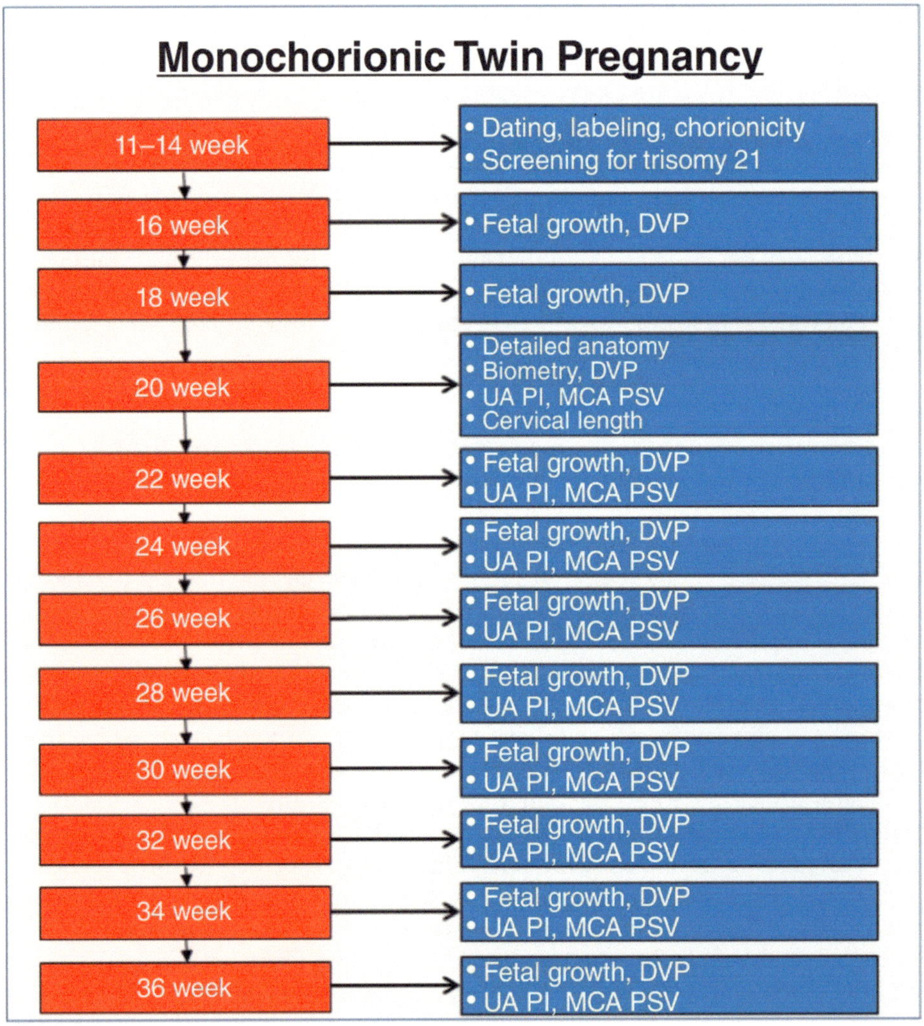

Figure 3.
Reproduced from Google image (Cambridge University Press).

At 16 and 18 weeks scan, it is recommended to measure foetal biometry and deepest vertical pocket (DVP) of amniotic fluid in each twin. At 20 weeks, a detailed anomaly scan should be performed along with biometry. The umbilical artery Doppler pulsatile index (UA PI) should also be recorded from this visit onwards along with the middle cerebral artery peak systolic velocity (MCA PSV). The MCA PSV helps in the early diagnosis of twin anaemia polycythaemia syndrome (TAPS) and is recommended to be done routinely from 20 weeks onwards [5]. Amniotic fluid measurements should be continued at this visit and a cervical length screening is also recommended at this stage. Antenatal visits should continue every 2 weeks until 36 weeks. At each visit, foetal biometry, umbilical artery Dopplers, middle cerebral artery peak systolic velocity and deepest vertical pocket of amniotic fluid in each sac should continue. A decision on delivery should be taken at 36 weeks.

8. Screening for structural anomalies

Twin foetuses should be assessed for the presence of any major anomalies at the first-trimester scan, and a routine second-trimester (anomaly) scan should be performed at around 20 (18–22) weeks of gestation as in singleton pregnancy.

Apart from this, a cardiac screening assessment should be performed in monochorionic twins. The cardiac scan should be performed according to standard ultrasound guidelines including laterality, situs and four-chamber, ventricular outflow tract and aortic arch. The abnormalities of the brain and cardiac abnormalities are more common in monochorionic twins. Other abnormalities associated with twins include neural tube defects, anterior abdominal wall defects, facial clefts, brain abnormalities, cardiac defects and gastrointestinal anomalies. Every 1 in 15 monochorionic pregnancies may have a risk of a major congenital anomaly. By doing a regular screening, the parents get a chance to prepare for the birth of a baby with a potential problem, offering them the option of termination. This also allows the transfer of the pregnancy to a tertiary care with special intervention facilities [5].

9. Screening for preterm birth

Cervical length assessment should be considered the optimal method of screening for preterm birth in a monochorionic pregnancy. A transvaginal scan visualises the cervix more objectively and the 2D modality is considered the most appropriate imaging modality.

The ratio of a curved/straight cervix decreases with a decrease in length, and this does not have important clinical implications [11]. Serial measurements should be done, and the shortest result should be taken. A short cervical length is a good predictor of preterm births even in later gestations. It is considered more accurate than digital exams and foetal fibronectin in the prediction of preterm birth (**Figure 4**) [12].

A cervical length of <20 mm at 20–24 weeks is the most accurate predictor of preterm labour with high sensitivity and specificity [12]. A higher rate of preterm birth is common in monochorionic twins and could be reflected and predicted by an increased rate of a short cervix.

The use of progesterone, bed rest, Arabin cervical pessary, antibiotics or oral tocolytics has not shown to reduce the risk of preterm labour in these cases. The use of vaginal progesterone in twin pregnancy with a TVS cervical length of <20–25 mm has

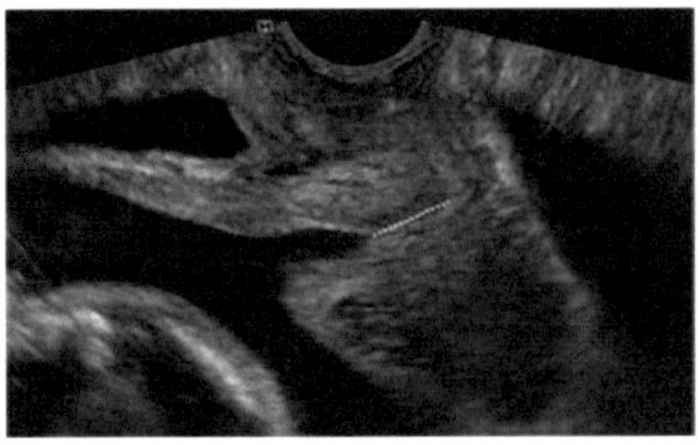

Figure 4.
Twin pregnancy with a short cervix. Courtesy: (mfmync.com).

been shown to reduce the incidence of preterm birth at <34 and <32 weeks in some studies [13]. However, the results were not conclusive. Progesterone may reduce the risk of neonatal morbidity and mortality [5].

The rates of preterm birth at <24 weeks, <28 weeks, <32 weeks and < 34 weeks have shown to be reduced by placement of a first-trimester cervical cerclage in twins only with a previous history of preterm birth [13].

A course of antenatal corticosteroids may reduce the risk of respiratory morbidity, necrotising enterocolitis and intraventricular haemorrhage but this should be timed and not given untargeted [14].

10. Screening and management of pathologies associated with monochorionic twins

10.1 Twin-to-twin transfusion syndrome

10.1.1 Aetiology

There is an increased number of arteriovenous (AV) anastomoses deep in the placenta in twin-to-twin transfusion syndrome. These are mainly capillary connections that happen in the cotyledon portion of the placenta. Unidirectional flow can occur in these AV anastomoses and result in shunting of blood towards one twin and away from the other, when the arteriovenous anastomoses are unbalanced. Bidirectional flow is usually maintained by arterioarterial (AA) and venovenous (VV) anastomosis. These are found more superficially on the placenta. AA anastomoses are thought to be protective against TTTS. There is apparently a reduction in AA anastomosis in monochorionic diamniotic twins and thus these twins are more susceptible to TTTS. On the other hand, monochorionic monoamniotic twins are thought to have more AA anastomoses, which is a theoretical reason why rates are lower in these twins than in MCDA twins [15, 16].

Due to the hypovolemia experienced by the donor twin, the renin-angiotensin-aldosterone system (RAAS) gets stimulated in that twin. This leads to oliguria and oligohydramnios. On the contrary, the other twin experiences hypervolemia which causes a cardiac stretch. This leads to an increase in atrial natriuretic peptide and brain natriuretic peptide release in the recipient twin. This inhibits the RAAS and leads to polyuria and polyhydramnios [17–19]. The consequences are atrioventricular valve insufficiency, diastolic dysfunction and pulmonary stenosis or atresia in the recipient twin.

Based upon data from referral centres, the Society for Maternal-Fetal Medicine (SMFM) estimates a prevalence of:

- Stage I: 11–15%
- Stage II: 20–40%
- Stage III: 38–60%
- Stage IV: 6–7%
- Stage V: 2% [20]

10.1.2 The diagnostic monitoring of TTTS

It is now well recognised that from 16 weeks onwards all women with monochorionic pregnancies should have a fortnightly ultrasound to diagnose TTTS. Literature suggests ultrasound-based signs as more reliable in the diagnosis of TTTS than physical examination or symptoms.

The ultrasound criteria recommended for the diagnosis of TTS are as follows:

Significant fluid discordance—this is very vital in the diagnosis of TTTS. An oligohydramnios with DVP less than 2 cm in the donor sac and polyhydramnios with a DVP greater than eight cm before 20 weeks and more than 20 cm after 20 weeks.

Discordant bladder appearances: No urine in the donor foetal bladder before 26 weeks of gestation. This should be used as a criterion of severe TTS.

Hemodynamic and cardiac comprise in both recipient and or donor twin [2].

Other studies suggest using hydrops fetalis (a condition associated with ascites, pleural, pericardial effusion and skin oedema) of the recipient twin as the criteria for ultrasound diagnostic features as well as growth restriction which can happen in 50% of donor twins as ultrasound criteria of TTTS along with the above standards. The foetal growth restriction is defined as an estimated foetal weight of <10% of normal or an abdominal circumference (AC) of <5% of normal in the setting of otherwise normal foetal growth [21].

10.1.3 Staging

The staging system is most utilised for TTTS is the Quintero Staging System, which is based upon two-dimensional ultrasound and Doppler study findings and is as follows:

- Stage I: oligohydramnios and polyhydramnios sequence, donor twin bladder is visible, Doppler studies of UA/UV/DV are normal in both twins.
- Stage II: oligohydramnios and polyhydramnios sequence, donor twin bladder is not visible, Doppler studies of UA/UV/DV are normal in both twins.
- Stage III: oligohydramnios and polyhydramnios sequence and abnormal Doppler study (only one of the following is required in either twin) [absent/reversed end-diastolic flow in UA, pulsatile flow in UV, or reversed a-wave flow in DV].

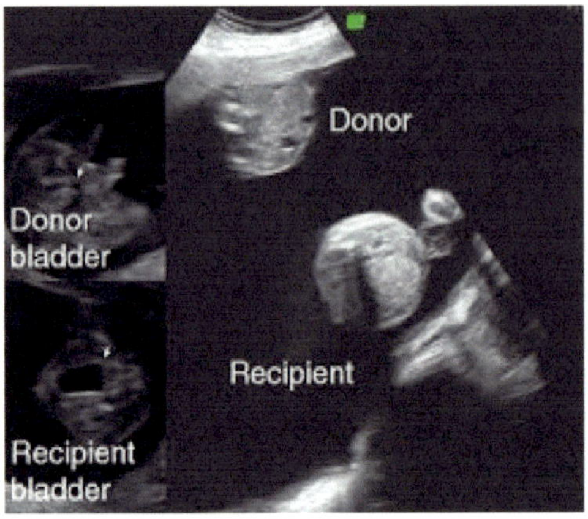

Figure 5.
Twin to twin transfusion syndrome. Courtesy (Springer open.com).

- Stage IV: oligohydramnios and polyhydramnios sequence, and one or both foetuses have hydrops.

- Stage V: oligohydramnios and polyhydramnios sequence, and one or both foetuses have died.

The above staging has been adopted from the Society of Maternal Fetal Medicine (**Figure 5**) [20].

10.1.4 Management options for TTTS

Management recommendations differ based on the stage of TTTS and gestational age and are outlined below [15].

- Stage I: The management of stage 1 is controversial. Expectant management is considered a recommended option. Similar outcomes comparing expectant management to amnioreduction and foetoscopic laser photocoagulation have been noted. Consider weekly ultrasounds for follow-up. Up to 25% of Stage I TTTS may progress to another stage. Expectant management is usually associated with a high survival chance of at least one twin in most pregnancies.

- Stage II, III, IV: The recommended treatment for these three stages is foetoscopic laser photocoagulation when the gestational age is <26 weeks. Laser photocoagulation has shown to have better outcomes than serial amnioreductions, including increased survival rates of one or both twins, delivery at greater gestational ages, and superior neurological outcomes. TTTS diagnosed before 26 weeks of gestation is best treated by laser ablation, as the evidence suggests that it leads to better outcomes compared with amnioreduction or septostomy. It is generally accepted that Quintero stages II and above will require treatment, and many centres will manage Quintero stage I conservatively. However, if laser ablation expertise is not available, amnioreduction is an acceptable alternative in pregnancies diagnosed after 26 weeks of gestation. There are some evidences that laser ablation is still the best form of treatment for TTTS, regardless of whether it is diagnosed early (before 16 weeks) or late (after 26 weeks of gestation).

- Stage V: No interventions have been evaluated at this stage.

Foetoscopic laser photocoagulation is the most well-known procedure for the management of TTTS. The rate of twin survival increases significantly after treatment with foetoscopic laser therapy up to 88% for at least one twin and 62% for the survival of both twins [22]. It should be performed under ultrasound guidance typically between 15 and 26 weeks of gestation. The aim of the procedure is to create 2 chorions which will individually supply blood to each twin. Although the procedure can be performed even earlier or later, there are drawbacks when performed at different times than recommended. If done below 16 weeks, the risk of PPROM is high while the risk of difficulty in coagulation exists after 25 weeks. This is mainly due to the increase in the size of blood vessels after 25 weeks.

The following are the various kinds of foetoscopic laser procedures used [23]:

A) Selective laser

In this procedure, at first, abnormal vessels are mapped by following them from origin to termination. A vessel that starts from one foetus, incorporates into a cotyledon and then journeys through the other foetus. This is considered pathologic, and it is this vessel which is photocoagulated. On the contrary, the vessel that leaves the cord as an artery, enters a cotyledon and returns to the same foetus as a vein is not pathologic and not treated. This procedure is called selective photocoagulation [21, 24].

Laser coagulation of the anastomoses is done through bursts of energy over 3–4 seconds from 1 cm. The laser energy can be tailored to the working distance, type and size of the vessels. If larger vessels are involved, multiple shots may be required to coagulate the vessels. Higher laser energy can be more efficient to prevent perforation of foetal vessels, bleeding and may lead to less placental damage. Typically (Nd: YAG: wavelenth 1066 nm are used).

Caution should always be taken to avoid contact between the laser fibre and tissue. In case, the targeted vessel is behind the membrane, the laser energy can be fired through the membrane.

B) Sequential laser

The coagulation in this procedure is done in the following way order of type of connections [21].

- Donor artery—recipient vein
- Recipient artery—donor vein
- Artery-artery
- Vein-vein
- AAs and VVs are usually called superficial anastomosis, whereas arteriovenous (AV) anastomosis typically involves an anastomosis between the artery and

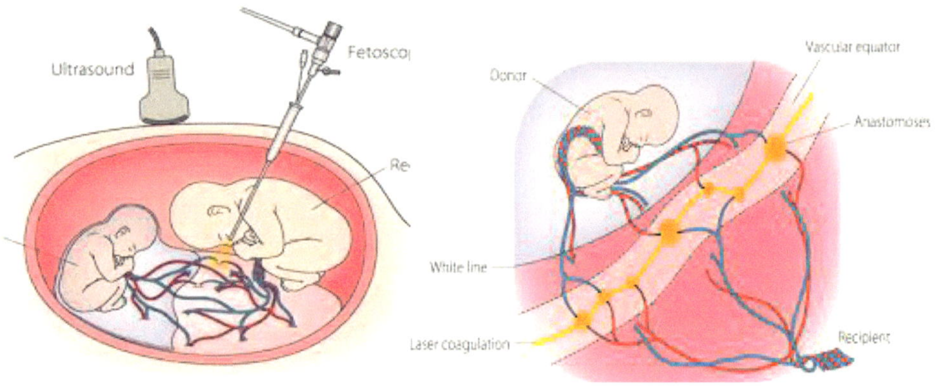

Figure 6.
Solomon technique: Courtesy—(google images-researchgate.net).

the vein and is called deep anastomosis. In an uncompensated case, the blood supply from the artery of one will twin will drain into the vein of the other twin. Sequential lasering involves grouped coagulation of AA, AV and VV anastomosis. In this technique, at first AV (donor to recipient) is coagulated, followed by VA (recipient to donor) [25]. Several studies (non-randomised) have shown better survival rates with this method. Technically, such a procedure reduces the risk of hypotension in the donor twin.

C) Solomon technique

The Solomon technique was developed as an advancement of coagulation techniques. The 'Solomon technique' involves initially completing coagulation of all visible anastomoses and then performing coagulation to connect the anastomoses ablation sites from one edge of the placenta to the other [22, 26]. This method enables the monochorionic placenta to be dichorionised by coagulating placental vessels and the surface of placenta. Although this technique results in fewer TTTS recurrences, decreased development of TAPS and increased perinatal survival, the risk of PPROM and placental abruption is high. This could be due to the increased exposure of the placental tissue to laser energy. This technique was found to be superior to the conventional technique in a randomised controlled study (**Figure 6**) [27].

10.1.5 Follow-up after laser coagulation

An initial follow-up a day after the procedure to rule out complications such as intrauterine death of one or both twins and cervical length.

The pregnancy can then be followed every two weeks as per the usual schedule. A weekly ultrasound is also recommended post-operatively [28]. The complications that could occur may be from procedure-related surgical complications to recurrences, brain, cardiac and limb abnormalities. As the procedure is associated with a risk of neurological damage, some centres perform a follow-up MRI, but this is still not a routine recommendation [27, 29].

Delivery is recommended in treated cases at around 35 weeks after giving steroids. Illustrative diagrams of various laser techniques (**Figures 7** and **8**).

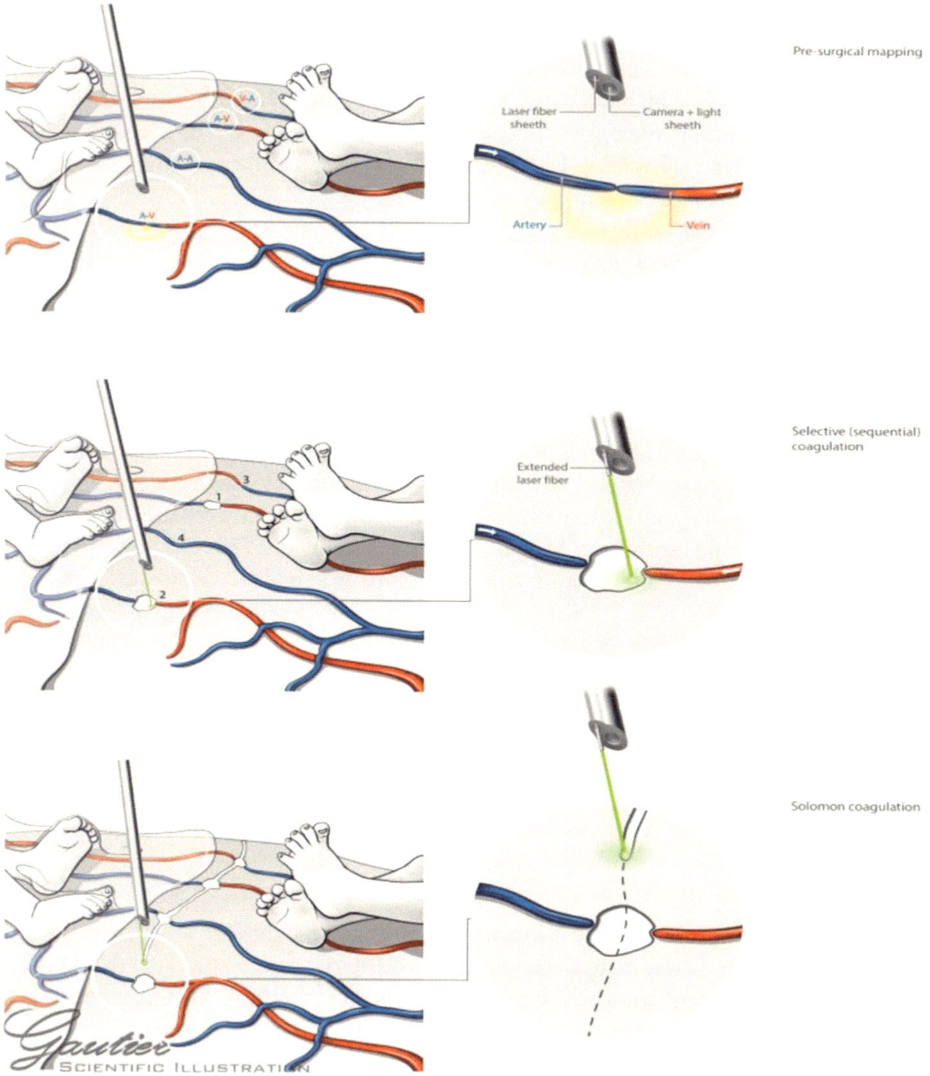

Figure 7.
Courtesy: Gautier Scientific Illustrations.

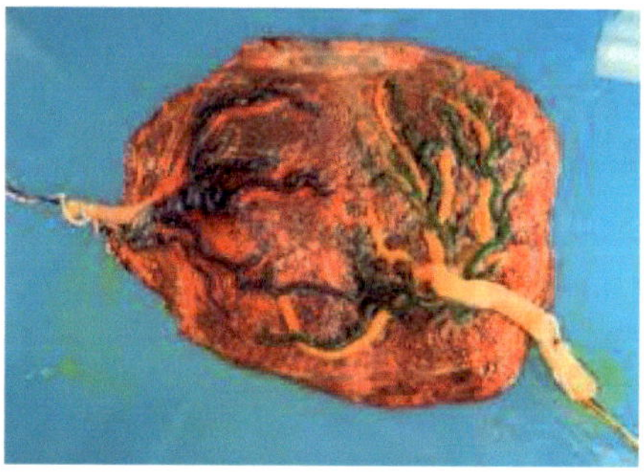

Figure 8.
Placental Anastomosis in TTTS (Courtesy: e-medicine.com).

10.1.6 Short- and long-term foetal outcomes following post laser treatment

Short-term early complications could include foetal demise of one or both twins. The risk is higher when the procedure is performed before 17 weeks. Similarly, the rates of preterm premature rupture of membranes (PPROM) may be higher when performed earlier than 17 weeks. TAPS may occur after missed small anastomosis in up to 3% of cases after dichoronisation.

Other complications could be a persisting or recurrent TTTS. This could happen in up to 1% of cases due to technical difficulties. A second laser could be a possibility but could be complicated by a haemorrhagic amniotic fluid due to a previous procedure.

Long-term foetal outcome shows that the survival of at least one or both twins is high. The survival rate of both twins is reported as 35–65%, whereas the survival of at least one twin is reported as between 70 and 88% [30]. Long-term neurodevelopment impairment was reported as 10% [31]. Neurological damage in TTTS may occur because of antenatal injury secondary to hemodynamic and haematological imbalance and/or from postnatal injury associated with prematurity [32] and low birth weight. Thermal injury damages may happen infrequently if unexpected foetal movements happen. A rare but serious complication could be vascular limb occlusion. This could vary from mild skin damage to total limb amputation and happens usually in the lower limbs.

10.1.7 Maternal complications of laser treatment

This could vary from mild peritoneal irritation due to leakage of fluid or blood in abdominal cavity, to other complications such as preterm labour, iatrogenic PPROM and delivery. Other complications could include infection, haemorrhage and placental abruption.

10.1.8 Amnioreduction

In the past, amnioreduction was the only treatment available for TTTS, but not anymore. Although foetal laser coagulation is now considered a gold standard for TTTS, a certain group of patients may still benefit from amnioreduction. Amnioreduction is also a more suitable option when TTTS is diagnosed after 26 weeks of gestation.

Amnioreduction is useful in the setting of TTTS when the criteria for laser surgeries are not met and when laser surgery is not technically possible in certain cases and in some cases of post-laser coagulation is a relatively simple treatment which does not require high-tech equipment [32].

Reduction of elevated amniotic fluid volume in polyhydramnios decreases the amniotic pressure which may lead to increased flow from the placenta to the foetus, as well as increases placental perfusion provided all other characteristics are unchanged. Controlled amnioreduction is considered a better option than random drainage of amniotic fluid [33].

Complications could include PPROM, infections, death of one or both twins (survival rates following this procedure range from 50 to 65%), need for serial amnioreductions, preterm labour, placental abruption, infection and decreased success of potential future foetoscopic laser photocoagulation [15]. The neurological impairments associated with amnioreduction are comparable with foetal laser therapy indicating that the predictor for neurological impairment is gestational age irrespective of management [32].

10.1.9 Septostomy

Septostomy is a procedure when an intentional rupture of the intertwin septum is done under ultrasound guidance. The aim of the procedure is to balance the amniotic fluid pressure in the two sacs. This may lead to a correction of the placental circulation, mainly in the donor twin's vessels. As the amniotic sac of the donor twin is filled, it reduces cord compression and improves foetal haemodynamics. As a result, the urine production of donor twin is improved [34].

Complications of septostomy are same as for serial amnioreduction, such as preterm labour and premature rupture of membranes. An additional risk is represented by the creation of a monoamniotic pregnancy that can lead to cord entanglement. The survival rates following septostomy for TTTS vary widely from 36 to 83%. Gestational age is increased in cases of septostomy compared with amnioreduction. Survival rates between septostomy and amnioreduction are comparable and septostomy offered the advantage of requiring a single procedure [34]. Another potential risk associated with septostomy is the presence of membrane flaps which may induce an amniotic band syndrome, a potentially dangerous complication. Experience with septostomy is limited and there is a need for further evaluation of this technique (**Figure 9**).

10.2 Twin anaemia polycythaemia sequence

Twin anaemia polycythaemia sequence (TAPS) is defined by significant intertwin haemoglobin discordance. It does not have the amniotic fluid discordance that characterises twin-twin transfusion syndrome (TTTS) in monochorionic twin pregnancies. This difference clearly distinguishes TAPS from TTTS.

TAPS is a rare disorder and can occur spontaneously (3–5%) or following foetoscopic laser ablation for TTTS (13–15%). This complication is thought to result from chronic transfusion through very small placental anastomoses. The pathogenesis of TAPS is not known.

A small number of usually very tiny and mostly unidirectional, arteriovenous placental anastomoses are seen in this condition. TAPS that follow laser surgery is associated with a smaller number of recurrent placental anastomoses than when it occurs spontaneously. The slow, and likely low volume, blood transfusion, which does not

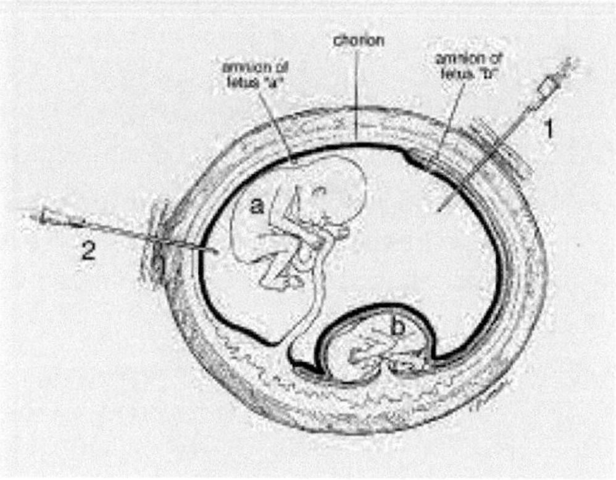

Figure 9.
Illustrative diagram of Septostomy (Courtesy: Semanticsscholar.org).

cause a great impact on the recipient's plasma volume (as the classic TTTS does), could be the possible explanation for there being no discordance in amniotic fluid volumes [35]. As a result of their extremely small size, these anastomoses can be missed during coagulation; thereby, Solomon technique is considered a better technique to prevent TAPS. The condition can be diagnosed both in antenatal and postnatal periods [36].

Middle cerebral artery peak systolic velocity (PSV) should be performed routinely following post-laser treatment to detect TAPS. The sensitivity of middle cerebral artery PSV to diagnose TAPS is more than 90%. Anaemia and polycythaemia both can be diagnosed using middle cerebral artery PSV antenatally. A middle cerebral PSV > 1.5 multiples of the median (MoM) for the donor twin and < 0.8 MoM in the recipient is proposed for antenatal diagnosis [37].

TAPS classification Antenatal stage Findings at Doppler ultrasound examination [37]:

- Stage 1—MCA-PSV donor >1.5 MoM and MCA-PSV recipient<1.0 MoM, without other signs of foetal compromise
- Stage 2—MCA-PSV donor >1.7 MoM and MCA-PSV recipient<0.8MoM, without other signs of foetal compromise
- Stage 3—as stage 1 or 2, with cardiac compromise of donor, defined as critically abnormal flow
- Stage 4—hydrops of donor
- Stage 5—intrauterine demise of one or both foetuses preceded by TAPS

Postnatal stage Intertwin Hb difference, g/dl

- Stage 1 > 8.0
- Stage 2 > 11.0
- Stage 3 > 14.0
- Stage 4 > 17.0
- Stage 5 > 20

Apart from the inter-twin haemoglobin difference of more >8 g/dl and one of the two following criteria should also be there; either a reticulocyte count ratio of >1.7 or the presence of only small vascular anastomoses (diameter 1 mm) on placental inspection (**Figure 10**) [37].

10.2.1 Treatment

Treatment options in utero include expectant management, intra-uterine transfusion both (intraperitoneal or intravascular) in the donor with or without partial exchange transfusion (PET) in the recipient, selective foeticide and laser therapy.

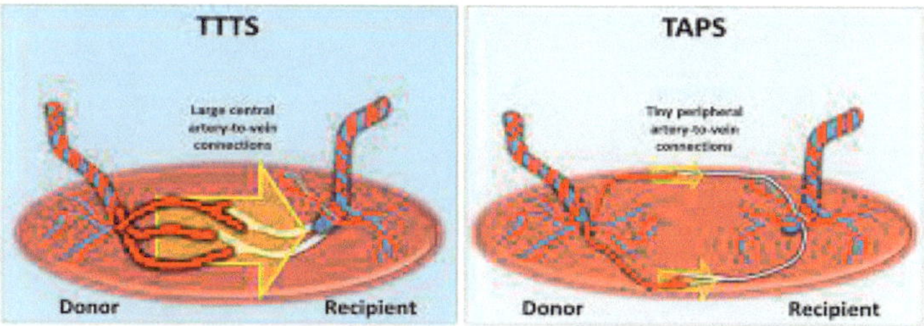

Figure 10.
The illustrative difference between TTTS and TAPS (courtesy—hopkinsmedicine.org).

Despite all options, laser remains the only treatment option that can resolve the possible causal mechanism. The preferred laser coagulation in TAPS should be the Solomon technique as this technique diminishes the risk of residual anastomoses and recurrent TAPS [38].

Intrauterine transfusions and partial exchange transfusions can temporarily stabilise the hemodynamic situation in severely affected foetuses. Overall, different management options may improve survival and perinatal outcomes like respiratory morbidities in affected foetuses [35, 39].

Some cases of intrauterine transfusions have been reported to be successful in prolonging the pregnancy. Even though the only pivotal treatment for TAPS is foetoscopic laser coagulation of the residue vascular anastomoses, this can be technically trickier than in TTTS. The reason for this is the absence of polyhydramnios and a stuck twin. This situation makes the visualisation of the vascular equator more difficult. The other reason is placental anastomoses in TAPS are known to be only few and minute. As a result, this may be missed during foetoscopy because of their size.

The precise perinatal mortality and morbidity frequency in TAPS is not known yet, probably because of the oddity of the condition. Spontaneous resolution of antenatal TAPS has also been described [40].

The results from recent studies suggest that spontaneous TAPS may have a better prognosis than post laser TAPS. As for mortality and morbidity, no differences were observed when comparing different management options for TAPS. Caution should be applied when interpreting these results due to scarcity of literature. A tailored antenatal management, considering the severity of TAPS and gestational age, is currently the recommended strategy [39].

10.2.2 Neonatal outcome

Haematological complications are commonly seen in TAPS donors and recipients. This may require postnatal blood transfusions or partial exchange transfusions. Another condition that the recipient can develop is polycythaemia hyper viscosity syndrome, which could possibly lead to necrosis of the skin and multiple limb ischemia. The recipient twin is also more at risk of thrombocytopenia due to impaired production because of tissue hypoxia [38].

Because of anaemia in donor twin and polycythaemia in recipient twin, cerebral injury can theoretically occur and cases of reported cerebral injuries have been reported in both twins. Recent studies show that long-term neurodevelopmental outcome in

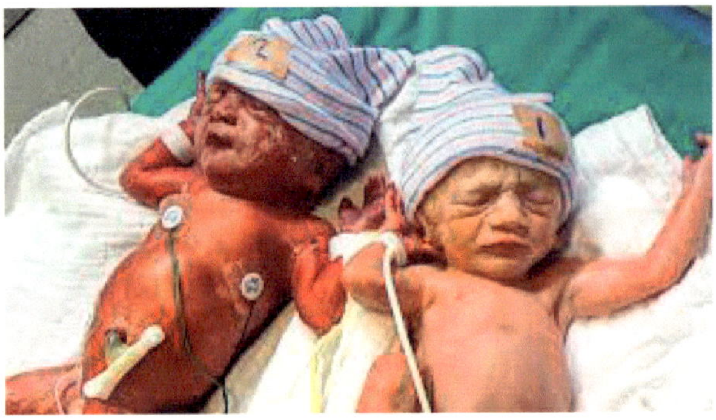

Figure 11.
Twin Anaemia Polycythaemia Syndrome—Courtesy:(en.wikepedis.org).

post-laser TAPS, not indicate mild to moderate cognitive delay in 9% and 17% of TAPS survivors, respectively. No difference in neurological impairment was found between donors and recipients. The rate of neurological impairment in TAPS seems to be comparable to the rate of impairment in children with TTTS after laser surgery. Risk factors may include early gestational age at delivery and smaller babies (**Figure 11**) [38].

10.3 Selective intrauterine growth restriction: (sIUGR)

This condition affects approximately 10–15% of monochorionic (MC) twin pregnancies. Selective intrauterine growth restriction is diagnosed when the estimated foetal weight (EFW) in one twin of <3rd percentile or an intertwin EFW discordance ≥25% is observed on ultrasound.

The main complications are the possible risk of intrauterine death of one twin or neurological damage of both twins. Unequal sharing of the placenta is the main cause of this condition, and the clinical outcome is closely related to the placental vascular anastomosis [41].

10.3.1 Pregnancy outcome in sIUGR:

- The risks of foetal demise of one or both foetuses
- Preterm delivery
- Subsequent development of TTTS
- Increased risk for neurodevelopmental impairment, with poorer outcome of the smaller twin

10.3.2 The diagnosis of sIUGR

Diagnosis of sIUGR is typically made in the second trimester based on foetal biometric measurements, growth discordance and umbilical artery (UA) Doppler parameters. sIUGR is defined as [42]:

- Estimated foetal weight (EFW) <3rd percentile of one foetus [5] or

- At least two of the four following criteria [42]:

- EFW <10th percentile for one twin

- Abdominal circumference < 10th percentile for one twin

- Weight discordance ≥25%

- UA pulsatility index >95th percentile for the smaller twin

It is recommended that from 20 weeks of gestation (at 2-weekly intervals) onwards at each scan the estimated foetal weight discordance should be calculated using two or more biometric parameters. The percentage EFW discordance should be calculated using the following formula:

([larger twin EFW – smaller twin EFW]/larger twin EFW) × 100. Liquor volumes as DVP should be measured and recorded (to differentiate from TTTS) [2].

As the EFW discordance of greater than 20% is associated with an increase in perinatal risks, these pregnancies should be referred to the specialist centres for further evaluation and management. One parameter that best reflects the differences in intrauterine growth restriction (IUGR) in monochorionic pregnancy with respect to singletons or dichorionic twins is umbilical artery (UA) Doppler flow. The characteristics of UA Doppler flow may be strongly affected by the existence of intertwin vascular connections.

In MC twin pregnancies complicated by sIUGR, UA Doppler waveforms represent the combined effect of placental insufficiency and placental vascular anastomoses.

Three main wave form patterns of diastolic flow in umbilical artery of smaller twin have been recognised. Hence, sIUGR is classified as [43]:

- Type 1—It is characterised by persistently forward UA end-diastolic velocity without variation in the waveform with normal or elevated resistance. This type has the best prognosis and the mean gestational age at delivery was after 35 weeks. It has the lowest risk of intrauterine foetal death and survival rates are high. Usually, late-onset sIUGR are type 1 and their prognosis is good as well, although they are at increased risk of TAPS.

- Type 2—It is characterised by fixed absent or fixed reversed UA end-diastolic velocity without any alteration of the waveform in the smaller twin. Affected foetuses will have worsening conditions in mid-trimester and the delivery is usually required at an average gestational age of 30 plus weeks.

Although pregnancies with type 2 sIUGR are anticipated to have a predictable pattern of deterioration and a longer latency period between diagnosis and deterioration than type 3 sIUGR, in terms of risk of death of one twin and preterm delivery, their prognosis is worst among all 3 types of sIUGR. Interestingly, there is usually no neurological damage seen in majority of survivors.

- Type 3—It is characterised by a pathognomonic UA waveform that has a variable flow pattern that cycles between forward, absent, and reversed flow over a short interval, which is termed intermittent absent/reversed end-diastolic flow. This happens due to a large artery-to-artery anastomosis on the placental surface and signifies the bidirectional volume flow across these vessels. It is more commonly observed in the UA of the smaller foetus since the interface of the two waveforms is shifted toward the smaller twin. An artery-to-artery anastomosis allows perfusion of oxygen and nutrients from the larger foetus to a portion of the smaller twin's placenta; consequently, type 3 sIUGR is associated with the largest degree of placental territory discordance (**Figure 12**) [44].

These pregnancies have unpredictable diagnosis, and foetal death can occur even shortly after a satisfactory ultrasound assessment. There is a high risk of neurologic morbidity as well, particularly of the larger twin. Survival rate has been reported up to 61%.

10.3.3 Diagnostic workup for suspected sIUGR should include

A detailed ultrasound anatomic survey of both twins to rule out structural anomalies.
Maternal viral serology or ultrasound markers to rule out foetal viral infections.
Evaluation of amniotic fluid of both twins to rule out coexisting TTTS and
Evaluation of middle cerebral artery peak systolic velocity to rule out coexisting TAPS.

10.3.4 Management based on the types

- sIUGR type 1—Expectant management

Weekly ultrasound surveillance of (umbilical artery [UA], middle cerebral artery [MCA]).

Weekly biophysical profile scoring (BPP) from 28 to 32 weeks.

If the UA pulsatility index increases to >95th percentile or the MCA pulsatility index falls below the 5th percentile, a twice weekly surveillance is recommended with additional monitoring of abnormalities in the ductus venosus (DV) waveform.

If foetal status remains reassuring, as it usually does, it is recommended to deliver delivery at 34 + 0 to 35 + 6 weeks (after steroids) as in pregnancies with sIUGR the risk of unexpected foetal death is higher than uncomplicated monochorionic pregnancies. Earlier delivery is indicated if deemed necessary for any maternal or foetal indications.

- sIUGR types 2 and 3—Due to the complexity of the condition the approach to these cases is more complicated. Death of one twin is high in these cases and can result in acute foetal transfusion and volume shifts, which leads to the double foetal demise or neurologic damage in the surviving co-twin in up to 30% of cases.

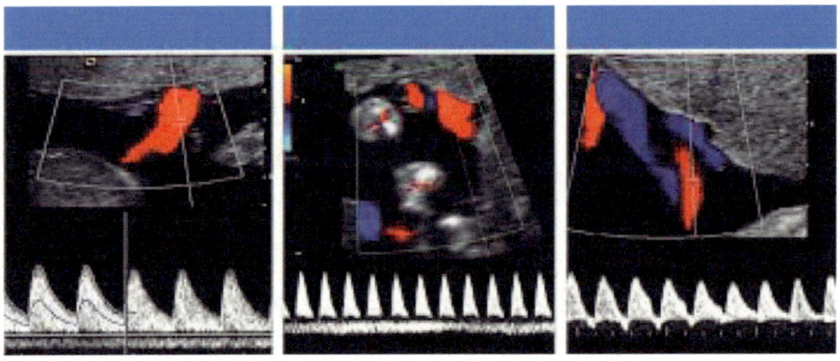

Figure 12.
The three types of selective intrauterine growth restriction (courtesy: isug.org).

The recommended approach may include either selective foetal reduction or foetoscopic laser ablation of intertwin placental vascular anastomoses (before the lower limit of viability), especially when there is foetal deterioration (progression from type 2 to type 3 sIUGR, venous Doppler abnormalities or oligohydramnios in the growth-restricted foetus.

Foetoscopic laser ablation can result in high mortality rate of the smaller twin and does not guarantee the survival of the normal twin but may protect the normally grown twin from the consequences of co-twin demise. The procedure may be more technically challenging compared with foetoscopic laser ablation for the treatment of twin-twin transfusion syndrome.

10.3.5 In patients not willing for above procedures

Weekly Doppler surveillance of UA, MCA and DV should commence from the diagnosis.

Perform weekly biophysical profile (BPPs) at 28 weeks.

If Doppler findings remain stable and BPPs are reassuring, they can be followed up as outpatients on a weekly basis.

If Doppler findings worsen increase surveillance with Dopplers/BPP to two to three times weekly and advise hospital admission for daily foetal monitoring with nonstress tests. Delivery should be considered between 32 and 34 week and earlier if indicated. Steroids should be given prior to deliver.

10.4 Selective feticide of one twin

Selective foeticide in monochorionic twins is performed by cord occlusion, intra-foetal laser ablation or radiofrequency ablation. The risk of miscarriage and or preterm birth may be influenced by the timing. A higher risk of these complications occurs when the procedure is performed in second trimester. When the diagnosis is made in the second trimester, a late selective termination in the third trimester can be offered to the woman, as the law permits. The risk of preterm birth in third trimester is less compared to the risk in second trimester. For selective foeticide of one twin of a monochorionic pair injection of intracardiac potassium chloride is not an option (unlike in dichorionic twin) due to the risk involved to the healthy co-twin. Instead, cord occlusion, intra-foetal laser ablation or radiofrequency ablation should be done. This procedure does not cause the healthy twin to lose its circulating blood volume in the terminating twin. The survival rate of the co-twin is approximately 80% in such cases [5].

Risks involved are:

- Premature rupture of the membranes and preterm birth in up to 20% of cases prior to 32 weeks.
- Miscarriages in second trimester.
- Increased risk of neurological damage in surviving twins.

10.5 Single intrauterine foetal demise. (Death of a co-twin)

Single intrauterine foetal demise (sIUFD) is a rare but exceptional perinatal problem in twin pregnancies. Monochorionicity and gestational age at the time of stillbirth seem to be decisive factors in terms of long-term neurologic outcome prediction for the survivor [45]. Monochorionic pregnancies are at particular risk of sIUFD due to bidirectional inter-twin placental vascular anastomoses. The intertwin blood flow becomes unbalanced and can lead to acute and chronic inter-twin transfusion and profound anaemia secondary to foetal exsanguination into the low-pressure circulation of the dead foetus [42]. The co-twin is at increased risk of preterm delivery, long-term neurological complications, and death especially when the condition occurs after 14 weeks of gestation.

The increased risk of neurological damage in the surviving twin could be due is to the bidirectional inter-twin vascular anastomoses that are found in monochorionic placentation. This results in unbalanced inter twin blood flow and leading to acute and chronic inter-twin transfusion and profound anaemia, which are seen in conditions such as TTTS, twin-anaemia-polycythaemia sequence (TAPS) and twin-oligo-polyhydramnios sequence (TOPS) [42]. As a result of these conditions, a multi-organ injury may occur causing significant hypoperfusion of the surviving twin. This may have been initiated by acute foetal exsanguination leading to low-pressure circulation of the dead foetus. The end results are hypoxic-ischaemic injury to the central nervous system of the surviving twin (up to 36%) and subsequent brain injury, or intrauterine death of the surviving twin [42, 46]. The other proposed theory is that "thromboplastic materials" from the dead twin to the surviving twin through the placental anastomosis which in turn causes disseminated intravascular coagulation (DIC) in the surviving twin. This results in renal, pulmonary, hepatic, splenic and neurological infarcts in surviving twin. But there are doubts as to the fact that the DIC can occur so fast; hence, it may be unlikely to be a causative mechanism [47].

10.5.1 Diagnosis

The most accurate diagnosis can be made by Magnetic resonance imaging (MRI). Diffusion weighted imaging (DWI) has recently been shown to add to the accuracy of the diagnosis with a timelier diagnosis [45].

Ultrasound detection of brain damage is possible in later stages of foetal brain injury. Also, ultrasound lesions may identify lesions like atrophic and necrotic cystic lesions or ventriculomegaly but not those associated with hypoxic ischemic injuries. This is due to the technical difficulty of the acoustic bone shadowing of skull bones. An early diagnosis and multidisciplinary counselling must be provided to the parents to make an informed choice.

Three types of injuries have been identified:

1. Ischemic hypoxic lesions of white matter which is irrigated by middle cerebral artery.

This leads to porencephaly, multicystic encephalomalacia, microcephaly and hydranecephaly.

2. Haemorrhagic lesions isolated or associated with ischemic lesions leading to post haemorrhagic hydrocephalus.

3. Anomalies secondary to vascular disruption leading to neural tubal defects and optic nerve hypoplasia.

The best time to identify these injuries on MRI is usually considered between 1 and 3 weeks. The use of DWI is unanimously accepted as superior with respect to the precocity of diagnosis. DWI signal changes occurring in cerebral ischemia may be detected early, within the first day of co-twin demise. Its usefulness is restricted to the first week after the death of the co-twin, interval after which pseudo normalisation occurs [45]. Decision to terminate pregnancy should be reserved for foetuses with severe ischemic injury (**Figure 13**).

10.5.2 The ethical and clinical challenges

A multidisciplinary team with maternal foetal medicine specialist, neonatologist, paediatric neurologist and neurosurgeon should be involved in counselling. Parents should be given accurate information to make a final decision. Should parents opt for continuing the pregnancy the risks of cerebral palsy and iatrogenic preterm delivery should be explained. Foeticide is not legally accepted in all countries. Social, cultural, and religious beliefs also add up in deciding.

10.5.3 Management

Management of such cases will also depend upon any maternal or foetal infections or conditions that could impair the survival of the other twin. DIC could also happen in rare cases because of the release of tissue thromboplastin from dead foetus in maternal circulation activating extrinsic coagulopathy. However, this is not very common (25%). As it occurs usually 3–5 weeks following foetal demise, clotting profiles should be performed in week 1 and repeat in 2–3 weeks [48].

In the short term, the surviving twin should be assessed for evidence of ongoing foetal compromise using CTG or MCA Doppler to assess for foetal anaemia. If conservative management is chosen, foetal biometry and assessment of umbilical and MCA Doppler should be scheduled every 2–4 weeks. Delivery should be considered at 34–36 weeks, after a course of maternal steroids. If the MCA-PSV is normal in the first few days, foetal anaemia is unlikely to occur later [5].

10.6 Twin Reversed Arterial Perfusion (TRAP)

Twin reversed arterial perfusion (TRAP) sequence, also named as acardiac malformation, is an exclusive complication of monochorionic multiple pregnancy. In this condition, one of the twins has no cardiac structure (and so is called 'acardiac'), while a morphologically normal co-twin (called 'pump twin') supplies both circulations. Historically, the first case was described by Benedetti in 1533, and the first cases

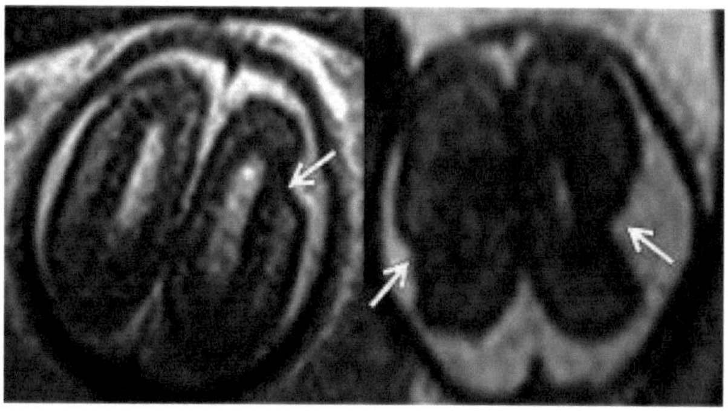

Figure 13.
MRI changes in the brain of the surviving twin after the death of co twin. Courtesy-(pubs.rsna.org).

had been reported in the international literature in the 1950s; the first description of prenatal diagnosis of an acardiac twin was reported by Lehr and Dire in 1978 [49].

10.6.1. Pathogenesis

Pathogenesis involves two pathways. First is that an unequal blood flow between the twins is noticed. The pump twin predominates due to its high-pressure flow, while the perfused twin receives a reversed deoxygenated blood flow. This leads to compromised morphogenesis. As there is no functioning heart developed the acardiac twin relies on the circulation of pump twin in a parasitic fashion.

The second pathogenesis proposed is that there is an embryogenic defect with a failure in heart formation, due to chromosome abnormality or environmental factors. Hence the single perfusion support for the acardiac foetus is received through anastomoses between the umbilical vessels. The acardiac twin is not viable but keeps getting vascular support from the pumped twin, which supplies deoxygenated blood to the acardiac twin. It has a well-developed body and upper extremities and a big size; hence, it remains a danger during the intrauterine period and is dangerous for the whole pregnancy.

The well-being of the pump twin can also be compromised through at least three mechanisms [49]:

1. Congestive heart failure (30%) and polyhydramnios of the pump twin (40%0, caused by a risen cardiac work due to the increased blood flow.

2. Preterm premature rupture of membranes (pPROM), preterm labour and preterm delivery (90%), caused by uterine overdistension, since the acardiac twin is often bigger than pump twin and it can reach a considerable size (acardiac twin to pump twin ratio > 70%).

3. Hypoxia and intrauterine growth restriction of the pump twin, caused by the deoxygenated blood that comes back to the pump twin through vascular anastomosis.

The perinatal mortality rate of this twin is 55%. The risk of demise of the pump twin in TRAP sequence if managed conservatively is up to 30% by 18 weeks.

10.6.2 Diagnosis

The diagnosis is made by ultrasound. Features noticed on ultrasound are:

a. Gross discrepancies in biometrical measurements of twins, regarding abdominal circumference.

b. Absence of a morphologically normal heart in one twin associated with several other malformations in head, trunk, upper and lower extremities: presence of subcutaneous oedema and fluid collections in the anomalous twin (**Figure 14**) [49].

Based on the morphology of the acardiac foetus, 4 different types have been described: acardiac acephalus; acardiac anceps; acardiac acormus; acardiac amorphous. However, they have no prognostic value and no difference in management options.

A classification based on prenatal ultrasound findings as acardius size and signs of impaired cardiac function of the pump twin have been proposed.

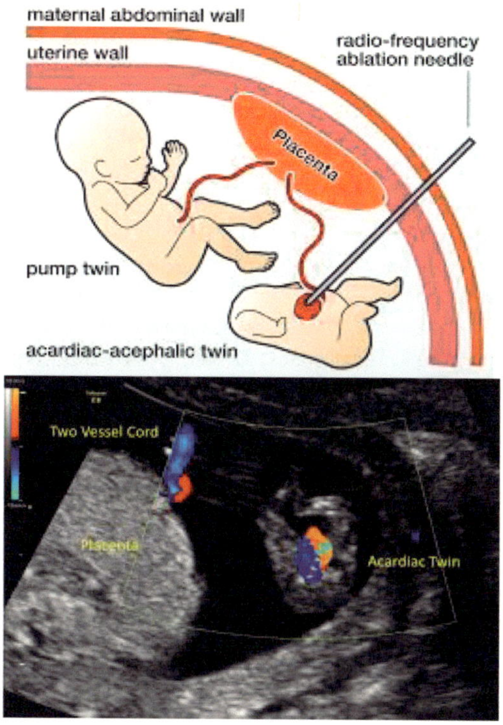

Figure 14.
Illustrative and ultrasound images of TRAP (courtesy—google image).

This classification may help in identifying the most severe cases and those that need prenatal interventions [49].

Acardiac anomalies are divided into:

- Type I: small or medium-sized acardiac twins, identified by an abdominal circumference ratio < 50%.
- Type II: large acardiac twins, in which the abdominal circumference ratio is ≥50%.

Each type can be further divided into a 'subtype a and b', if pump-twin does not show signs of cardiovascular failure, or into a subtype.

10.6.3 Management

The main goals in the management of the TRAP sequence are preserving the survival of the pump twin and reaching the term for delivery. It is observed that the prognosis of the pump twin in Type Ia, acardiac foetus is quite reassuring. This allows a conservative management of pregnancy through periodic ultrasound. This approach is associated with a good outcome in 88% of cases. In the presence of an acardius Type Ib, it is reasonable to repeat ultrasound to identify a spontaneous resolution or a worsening that requires invasive treatment.

The Type IIa acardiac foetus can be large because of subcutaneous oedema or hydrops, and even if now of diagnosis, the pump foetus shows no signs of cardiac failure, the large size could threat the whole pregnancy due to an increased risk of preterm labour. In this case, a prenatal treatment is required. The detection of a Type IIb acardius requires a prompt intervention [49].

The best timing of intervention is not clear. It should be performed preferably before 16 weeks [5]. A pump-twin loss rate of 33% in the time elapsed from the first-trimester diagnosis and the elective intervention at 16–18 weeks, highlights an important disadvantage of delayed intervention. A multicentre, open-label, randomised controlled trial currently ongoing (ClinicalTrails.gov: NCT02621645), named the TRAP Intervention Study (TRAPIST), comparing treatment at 13–15 weeks vs. treatment from 16 weeks, is expected to define the optimal timing of treatment.

Different minimally invasive techniques, such as cord coagulation, cord ligation and photocoagulation of the anastomoses, as well as intrafoetal methods, such as Radiofrequency Ablation and intrafoetal laser therapy, are performed as a means of preventing the demise of the pump twin. The survival rate of the pump twin using these treatment modalities is approximately 80%. TRAP sequence pregnancies should be monitored serially. The aim is to take intrauterine therapy as an option if cardiac strain becomes evident in the pump twin or there is increased perfusion (including the occurrence of polyhydramnios) and growth of the TRAP mass. Hence, these cases should be managed in a tertiary level centre [5].

11. Timing of delivery and Intrapartum management of uncomplicated monochorionic twins

Parents should be informed that usually a planned birth is recommended at 36 completed weeks and this does not increase the risk of any neonatal morbidity [10]. It is well documented that continuing pregnancy beyond 36 weeks is associated with increased risk of still births in monochorionic pregnancies. With an uncomplicated monochorionic twin pregnancy, vaginal birth and planned caesarean section are both safe choices for them, and vaginal delivery can be offered if the following criteria are met [10]:

- The pregnancy was uncomplicated throughout and has progressed beyond 32 weeks.

- There are no obstetric contraindications to labour.

- The first baby is in a cephalic (head-first) presentation.

- There is no significant size discordance between the twins.

If the first twin is not cephalic at the time of birth, a caesarean section should be offered. Corticosteroids should be offered prior to the planned delivery at 36 weeks.

During labour continuous, cardiotocography (CTG) should be commenced. A dual channel cardiotocography monitor should be used to allow simultaneous monitoring of both foetal hearts. As labour progresses, a foetal scalp electrode can be used for the first twin if no contraindications. If there is foetal dress and foetal blood sampling cannot be done, caesarean section should be performed after the birth of the first baby.

Once the first twin is delivered, continue to monitor the second baby using CTG. If the CTG shows a 'suspicious' or 'pathological' pattern, and vaginal birth is not possible within 20 minute a caesarean section should be offered. Epidural should be offered for vaginal birth and regional anaesthesia for caesarean section.

Third stage should be managed actively with controlled cord traction and oxytocin (Active management). In a vaginal birth, active management consists of 10 IU of oxytocin by intramuscular injection immediately after the birth of the last baby and before the cord is clamped and cut. In a caesarean section, it consists of 5 IU of oxytocin by intravenous injection immediately after the birth of the last baby and before the cord is clamped and cut [10].

12. Conclusion

MCDA twins are associated with several well-known complications. Updated guidelines and basic standards should be adhered to for a better outcome of these complications. Challenging cases may need individual care, but basic principles of early screening, diagnosis, accurate follow-up, and timely intervention should be the best approach. Poor or suboptimal care may directly be related to lack of observance to updated guidelines and non-accessibility of advances in management. The advanced role of ultrasound and relatively newer technologies such as laser photocoagulation for the treatment of severe TTTS, radiofrequency ablation and cord occlusion for selective reduction have significantly enhanced the outcomes for many of the complications of MCDA twins. Screening for these conditions is of paramount significance for the early diagnosis with timely intervention to improve neonatal morbidity and mortality. A first-trimester ultrasound to evaluate the interface of the intertwin membrane with the placenta, timely detection of chorionicity and antenatal surveillance of these pregnancies is the key to improved outcomes in MCDA twins. Future researches are required to further improve the overall survival rate and reduce the incidence of neurological impairment associated with intervention procedures.

Author details

Rafiea Jeddy[1,2]

1 Department of Obstetrics and Gynaecology, Royal College of Ireland, Bahrain

2 American Mission Hospital, Bahrain

*Address all correspondence to: rjeddy@rcsi.com

References

[1] Gill P et al. Twin Births-STAT PEARL-NCBI Bookshelf. Stat Pearls Publishing. Last updated-May11,202. Available online: http://www.ncbi.nlm.nih.gov/books/NBK493200

[2] Monochorionic Twin Pregnancy Management. Green top Guideline No 51,RCOG. Available online: http://www.rcog.org.uk>guidance>green-top-guidelines

[3] Denbon ML et al. Placental angioarchitecture in monochorionic twin pregnancy, relationship to fetal growth, feto fetal transfusion and Pregnancy Outcome-American. Journal of Obstetrics and Gynaecology. 2000;**182**:417-426

[4] Karim M, Mary ED. Alton-Chorioncity of Multiple Gestation. ELSEVIER. Obstetric Imaging. Fetal Diagnosis and Care. Second Edition; 2018. p. 639-641

[5] International Society of Ultrasound in Obstetrics and Gynaecology (ISUOG). Practice Guidelines: Role of Ultrasound in Twin Pregnancy. Wiley online library.com

[6] Lee SW et al. Clinical utility of increased nuchal translucency in twin pregnancy based on chorionicity. Journal of Clinical Medicine. 2021

[7] Linskens I, et al. Discordance in nuchal translucency measurements. American Journal of Obstetrics and Gynaecology. Twin Research And Human Genetics. Cambridge University Press,21/2/2021. 2008;**12**(6):605-610

[8] Cheng Y et al. Performance of non-invasive prenatal testing for fetal chromosomes in 1048 pregnancies. Molecular Genetics. 2021;**32**

[9] International Journal of Gynaecology and Obstetrics. Mar 2019;**144**(3):330-337. DOI: 10.1002/ijgo.12742

[10] Twin and Triplet Pregnancy |Guidance. NICE guideline. Published 4 September 2019. Available online: www.nice.org.uk/guidance/ng137.

[11] Brigut A. Prevention of preterm delivery in twins. prenatal. Cardiology. 2014;**4**:5-12

[12] Roman A et al. Mid trimester cervical length screening for preterm birth in diamniotic twin pregnancy according to chorionicty. European Journal of Obstetrics Gynaecology Reproductive Biology. 2;**229**:57-63

[13] Amanda et al. Prevention of preterm birth. Expert Review. 2021;**4**:100551

[14] Roberts et al. Antenatal steroids for accelerating fetal lung maturity for females at risk of preterm birth. Cochrane Data Systematic Reviews. 2006;**3**:CD004454

[15] Borse V, et al. Twin to twin transfusion syndrome. National Library of Medicine; Stat Pearls Publishing. May 1,2022 . Available online: http://www.ncbi.nlm.nih.gov./books/NBK563133

[16] Bamberg C. K-Update on twin to twin transfusion syndrome. Best Practices Research in Clinical Obstetrics and Gynaecology. Jul 2019;**58**:55-65

[17] Mahicu Caputo D et al. Twin to twin transfusion syndrome-role of fetal renin angiotensin system. American Journal of Pathology. 2000;**156**(2):629-636

[18] Barjoria R et al. Influence of vasopressin in the pathogenesis of oligo/polyhydramnios in MC twins. European

Journal of Obstetrics and Gynaecology. 2004;**113**:49-3655

[19] Barjoria R et al. Natriuretic peptide in pathogenesis of cardiac dysfunction in recipients of TTTS. American Journal of Obstetrics and Gynaecology. 2002;**186**:121-127

[20] Simpson L. L-twin to twin transfusion syndrome. American Journal of Obstetrics and Gynaecology. 2013;**208**:3-18

[21] Garth E. Fletcher-Medscape Practice Essentials. 2019

[22] Akkermans J et al. What is the impact of placental tissue damage after laser surgery for TTTS-A secondary analysis of Solomon Trial. Placent. 2017;**52**:71-76

[23] Van Der Veekan L et al. Laser for twin to twin syndrome. A guide to endoscopic surgeons. Facts, Views and Visions in Obstetrics and Gynaecology. 2019;**11**:197-205

[24] Quintero et al. Selective v/s nonselective laser photocoagulation of placenta vessels. Ultrasound Obstetrics Gynaecology. 2000;**16**(3):230-236. DOI: 10/1046/j.1469-0705.2000.00265

[25] Quintero et al. Sequential selective laser photocoagulation in TTTS. Journal of Maternal, Fetal and Neonatal Medicine. 2006;**20**:763-768

[26] Sago H et al. Fetoscopic laser photocoagulation for TTTS. The Journal of Obstetrics and Gynaecology Research. 2018;**44**:831-838

[27] Slagghekke et al. Fetal laser coagulation of the vascular equator v/s selective coagulation for TTTS. Lancet. 2014;**383**:2144-2151

[28] Khalil et al. Role of ultrasound in twin pregnancy. Ultrasound Obstetrics and Gynaecology. 2016;**47**:247-263

[29] Knijnerburg KGC et al. Incidence and risk factors for residual anastomosis in TTTS treated with Laser Surgery—A 15 year single centre experience. Fetal Diagnosis Therapy. 2017

[30] Akkermans et al. Laser coagulatin in TTTS. A systematic review. Fetal Diagnosis Therapy. 2015;**38**:241-253

[31] Van Klin JM et al. Long term neurodevelopmental outcome in survivors of TTTS-Twin. Research and Human Genetics. 2016;**19**(3):255-261. DOI: 10.1017/thg.2016.26

[32] Li X et al. Prognosis and long-term neurodevelopment outcome in conservatively treated TTTS. BMC Pregnancy and Child Birth. Article 32(2011). Available online: http://www:biomedcentral.com/1471-2393/11/32

[33] Gordon Z et al. Controlled amnioreduction. Research Article. Mar 29 2022;**16**

[34] A Cristina Rossi. Twin to Twin Transfusion Syndrome. Medscape CME and Education. Available online: http://www.medscape.org>viewarticle

[35] Moaddab A et al. TAPS, a single centre experience and literature review. European Journal of Ob/Gyn and Reproductive Biology. 2016;**265**:158-164

[36] Giorgiona V et al. Systematic reviews and meta analysis. Perinatal outcome complicated by TAPS. Ultrasound in Obstetrics and Gynaecology. 2021;**58**(6):813-823

[37] Slaghekkae F et al. TAPS, diagnostic criteria classification, perinatal management and outcome. Twin Research and Human Genetics;**19**(3):222-223

[38] Lisanne SA et al. TAPS. Current view on pathogenesis and diagnostic criteria. Twin Research and Human Genetics;**199**(3):222-223

[39] Sananes N et al. Evaluation of the utility of in utero treatment of TAPS. Fetal Diagnosis and Therapy. 2015;**38**(3):170-178. DOI: 10.1159/000380822

[40] Ayre K et al. Antenatal management of TAPS: A case report. Medical Science International Medical Journal. 2018;7(3):709-712

[41] Rustico MA et al. Selective IUGR in Monochorionic Twins. Changing Patterns in Umbilical Artery Doppler and Outcome. Ultrasound in Obstetrics and Gynaecology. Mar 2017;**49**(3):387-393

[42] Mackie F et al. Fetal Brain Injury in Survivor of Twin Pregnancy Complicated by Demise of One Twin. Twin Research and Human Genetics. Cambridge University Press. 2016;**19**(3):262-267. DOI: 10.1017/thg.2016.39

[43] Miller J et al. Selective fetal growth restriction in monochorionic twin pregnancy complicated by demise of one twin. Literature Review. 2021

[44] Gratacos et al. A classification system for selective IUGR in monochorionic pregnancy according to umbilical artery doppler in smaller twin. Ultrasound Obstetrics and Gynaecology. 2007;**30**:28-34

[45] Gheorghe L et al. Imaging diagnosis and legal implications of brain injury in survivors following single intra uterine demise from monochorionic twin. A review of literature. Perinatal Medicine. Apr 22, 2021;**49**(7):837-846

[46] Hillman et al. Cotwin prognosis of a single fetal death: A systematic review and metanalysis. Obstetric Gynaecology. 2011;**118**:928-940

[47] Hillman et al. Single twin demise. Consequences for Survivors. Seminars in Fetal and Neonatal Medicine. 2010;**15**:319-320

[48] Stefanescu BI et al. Single fetal demise in twin pregnancy: A great concern but still a favourable outcome. Diseases. 2021;**9**:33

[49] Vitucci et al. TRAP sequence: Current treatment options. International Journal of Womens Health. 2020;**28**:435-443. DOI: 10.2147/IJWH.S214254.2020

Section 3

Breastfeeding

Chapter 7

Perceived Insufficient Milk Supply (PIMS) in Lactating Mothers

Yakov Y. Yakovlev

Abstract

Perceived inadequate milk supply (PIMS) is a factor that hinders successful breastfeeding. The aim of our study was to determine the predictors of PIMS and to evaluate the effect of PIMS on the duration of lactation. More than 5000 mothers with children who had been breastfeeding for some time participated in our study. Analysis was performed using multivariate regression logistic and ROC statistical analyses. Eight predictors increasing the risk of PIMS were identified.

Keywords: breastfeeding, insufficient milk supply, lactation, perceived inadequate milk supply, PIMS

1. Introduction

Adequate breast milk intake by the baby and milk production by the mother can be compared to the paradox of "Which came first, the chicken or the egg?" What is primary, a decrease in milk consumption or a decrease in milk production? Does the deficiency of milk occur after the baby's intake decreases, or does the deficiency of milk lead to the decrease in intake? [1, 2].

In addition to the terms "not enough milk" and "insufficient milk," the literature mentions the terms "perceived insufficient milk," "insufficient milk supply," and "perceived insufficient milk supply," describing the same process—the feeling (perception) of not having enough milk [1–4]. Perceived insufficient milk supply (PIMS) is a mother's belief that she is not producing enough milk for her infant, when in fact there is no objective evidence of normal or low milk production [1, 3]. As a result of the suspicion of a lack of milk, breastfeeding mothers may introduce formula for complementary feeding without objective reasons, which negatively affects the continuation of breastfeeding. There are no Russian papers analyzing the causes of PIMS and their effect on lactation.

The aim of our study was to identify predictors of PIMS in breastfeeding mothers and to evaluate the effect of PIMS on the duration of exclusive breastfeeding (EBF) and breastfeeding (BF).

For the analysis, a sample of mother-child pairs whose data were obtained over a 20-year period in several surveys was formed. The mothers were interviewed using a paper questionnaire and an electronic questionnaire online. Informed consent to participate in the study was obtained from all respondents. At any time, participants could stop entering data, which was regarded as a refusal to participate. After processing 6595 questionnaires, the answers of 5414 mothers who lived in the Russian Federation and answered the question about the presence or absence of the PIMS problem were included in the work. Among all included mothers, 40.4% (2187/5414) had already completed breastfeeding and 59.6% (3227/5414) continued lactation. The data were obtained from more than 450 localities in the Russian Federation.

Statistical analysis of the obtained data was performed using licensed software STATISTICA 13RU. Missing data (absence of answer in the questionnaire) were excluded from statistical processing during the analysis. The level of statistical significance (p) for all statistical analysis procedures was calculated and 0.05 was accepted as critical. The character of quantitative variables distribution was determined by Shapiro-Wilk criterion. At $p < 0.05$, the null hypothesis of normal distribution was rejected. Most of the quantitative data in the study did not have a normal distribution. Therefore, the number of samples from the total number of subjects (n/N), median (Me), and interquartile range (Lower Quartile (LQ) = 25th and Upper Quartile (UQ) = 75th percentile) were used to describe these measures. Data are given as Me (LQ; UQ). Comparison of quantitative characteristics in the two independent groups with a non-normal distribution was performed using the Mann-Whitney U-criterion. A logistic regression model was used to identify and assess the significance and influence of predictors on the target binary variable. In the analysis, missing data were replaced by the mean and a quasi-Newtonian estimation method was used. Neural network ROC-analysis was used to analyze the quality of the models obtained. Estimation of risk (unfavorable outcome) or probability (favorable outcome) of any event in retrospective analysis was done using the ratio of chances of event in one group to the chances of the same event in the other group. Adjusted odds ratio (AOR [CI 95%]) was calculated in logistic regression, and unadjusted odds ratio (UOR [CI 95%]) was calculated when comparing other predictors. The censored data were evaluated with a survival function using the Kaplan-Meier procedure. The median time and quartiles of GW and IGW cessation were determined. Comparison of two samples with censored features was performed using Wilcoxon-Gehan criterion.

2. Study results

A history of PIMS was reported by 38.8% (2101/5414) of the 5414 mothers interviewed. This problem statistically significantly increased the risk of complementary feeding by a factor of 3.4 (OR = 3.36 [2.92; 3.87]). Maternal PIMS had a negative effect (**Figures 1** and **2**) on both the duration of EBF and the duration of BF. Among mothers with PIMS, the median duration of lactation was 4 months shorter than among mothers without the problem, 8 and 12 months, respectively ($p < 0.001$). The median duration of EBF was 1 month shorter at 5 and 6 months, respectively ($p < 0.001$).

All respondents were divided into two groups. The first "PIMS" group included 2101 mothers who indicated a history of PIMS at 2.0 (1.0; 3.0) months of age. The second "Control" group included 3313 mothers who did not indicate a history of PIMS.

Babies in the PIMS group were statistically significantly more likely to be first and from the first pregnancy, as well as those born by cesarean section (**Table 1**) compared with the control group. These predictors increased the risk of PIMS by 15.0, 19.0, and 40.0%, respectively. Paternal education was more common in the control group. However, all of these predictors were not included in the statistically significant PIMS risk model in the multivariate analysis.

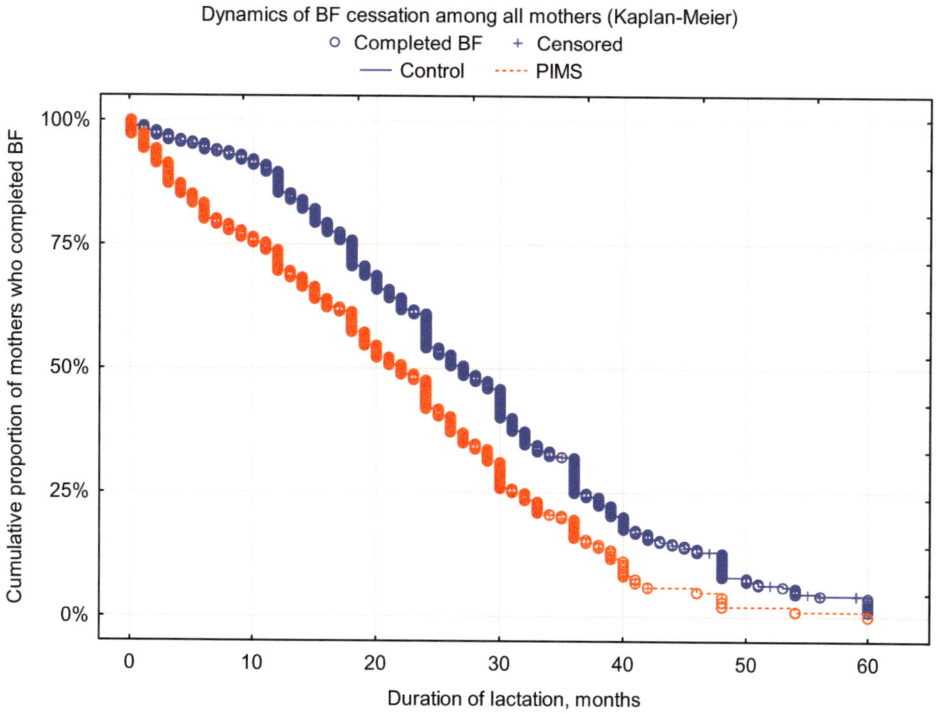

Figure 1.
Dynamics of BF cessation in mothers.

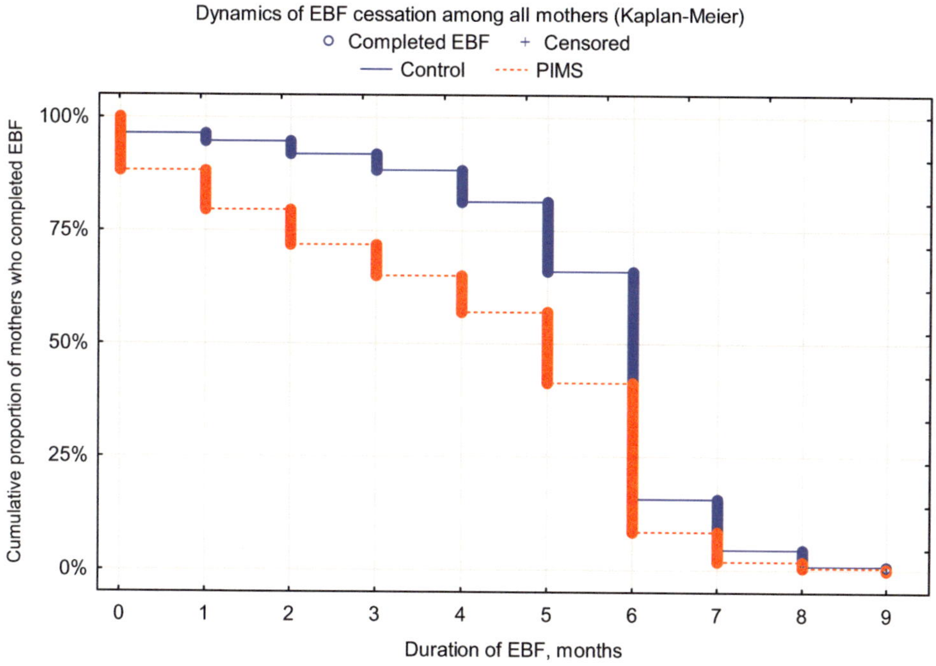

Figure 2.
Dynamics of EBF cessation in mothers.

Predictors	Group "PIMS", n = 2101, n/N (%)	Group "Control", n = 3313, n/N (%)	p	UOR [CI 95%]
First pregnancy	1226/2078 (59.0)	1815/3262 (55.6)	0.016	1.15 [1.03; 1.28]
First baby	1545/2090 (73.9)	2310/3280 (70.4)	0.006	1.19 [1.05; 1.35]
Cesarean section	460/1730 (26.6)	600/2930 (20.5)	< 0.001	1.40 [1.22; 1.61]
Higher education of the father	1480/2074 (71.4)	2430/3276 (74.2)	0.024	1.15 [1.02; 1.31]

Table 1.
Differences in predictors in comparison groups.

Age period	Group «PIMS», n = 2101, n/N (%)	Group "Control", n = 3313, n/N (%)	p
From 0 to 1 month	800 (500; 1060)	1025 (770; 1300)	< 0.001
From 1 to 2 months	950 (750; 1182)	1011 (840; 1300)	< 0.001
From 2 to 3 months	842 (658; 1000)	870 (700; 1070)	0.015

Table 2.
Dynamics of body weight gain in comparison groups.

Code of predictor	Predictors	β	Wald's Chi-square	p	UOR [CI 95%]	AOR [CI 95%]
	Constant (β_0)	–1.67		< 0.001		
p_1	Supplementary feeding with formula after discharge from the maternity hospital	0.91	132.02	< 0.001	3.36 [2.92; 3.87]	2.49 [2.13; 2.91]
p_2	Regular breast expressions	0.62	65.66	< 0.001	2.69 [2.35; 3.08]	1.86 [1.60; 2.16]
p_3	Separation of mother and baby up to 6 months of age	0.30	18.28	< 0.001	1.64 [1.44; 1.87]	1.35 [1.18; 1.55]
p_4	Supplementary feeding with formula in the maternity hospital	0.59	16.15	< 0.001	2.03 [1.55; 2.66]	1.80 [1.35; 2.40]
p_5	Late first latch	0.24	14.86	< 0.001	1.54 [1.38; 1.72]	1.27 [1.12; 1.43]
p_6	No prenatal preparation for breastfeeding	0.21	10.54	0.001	1.32 [1.17; 1.48]	1.23 [1.09; 1.40]
p_7	Water supplementation in the first half of the year	0.30	14.54	< 0.001	2.31 [2.02; 2.63]	1.35 [1.16; 1.57]
p_8	Maternal higher education	0.27	8.67	0.003	0.85 [0.73; 1.00]	1.30 [1.09; 1.56]

Table 3.
Logistic regression model of predictors.

Prematurity, sex of the baby, separation of mother and baby in the maternity hospital, desire to breastfeed in the woman, age of the parents and financial status in the family did not differ in frequency between the groups. They were also not included in the statistically significant probability model of PIMS and did not influence the risk of PIMS.

In the "PIMS" group compared with the "Control" group, children gained less statistically significantly at 2.0 (1.0; 3.0) months of age when milk deficiency was suspected (**Table 2**). However, these differences had no clinical significance.

A multivariate regression analysis using logistic regression was performed. A statistically significant ($p < 0.001$) model included eight of the 20 predictors (**Table 3**). The percentage of values correctly predicted by the model (diagnostic efficiency) was 66.31%, and the disagreement ratio was 3.35.

In the logistic model including the Chi-square Wald criterion, the most significant predictor with a negative effect was infant formula administration after the maternity hospital—this predictor increased the adjusted risk of PIMS by 2.5-fold. Other predictors increased the risk of PIMS from 1.23 to 1.86-fold, including lack of maternal education. The effect of the latter was statistically significant and increased the adjusted risk of PIMS by a factor of 1.3.

According to the results of ROC analysis, the model quality is good (AUC area 0.73), cutoff value 0.64 (**Figure 3**). The sensitivity of the test was 35%, specificity 86%, and diagnostic efficiency 66%.

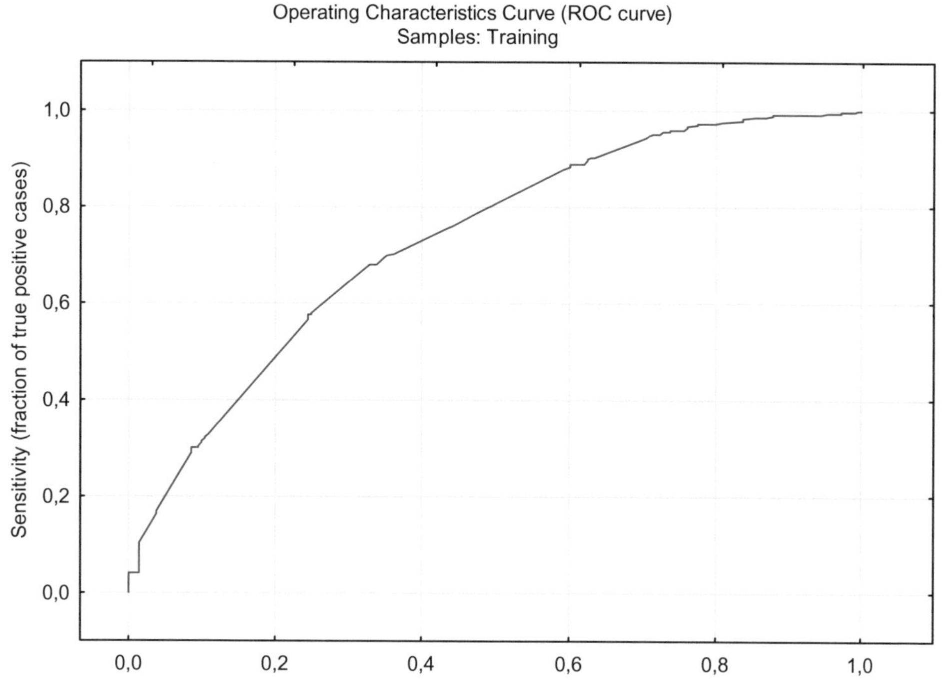

Figure 3.
ROC curve of the logistic model.

3. Discussion

Lactation is initiated during the first days after birth (lactogenesis II), when endocrine regulation of breast milk formation changes to autocrine regulation. The key point in this process is early first lactation, maximal mother-baby contact, and exclusive breastfeeding. The entire subsequent regulation of lactation (lactogenesis III) is related to the frequency and completeness of breast milk elimination from the lactocytes, which contributes to the adequate functioning of prolactin receptors and a decrease in the accumulation of lactation feedback inhibitor in the mammary gland. Frequent lactation and nipple stimulation suppress the production of prolactin-inhibitory factor in the hypothalamus, including by reducing the production of dopamine. The presence of factors negatively affecting lactogenesis II and lactogenesis III at any stage of development or during the established lactation leads to a decrease in the duration of BF [1, 2, 5].

In 2008, Lisa Gatti, in a published literature review, described PIMS in 30–80% of mothers, especially those who stopped breastfeeding early in the absence of objective signs of hypogalactia [3]. According to this review, PIMS ranks as one of the leading causes of lactation cessation. Also, the literature suggests that PIMS is an ongoing risk throughout lactation [3]. In other sources, the causes and predictors of PIMS are not fully reflected, are not systematic, and the exact prevalence of the problem among nursing mothers is not known [1, 2].

In our study of 5414 mothers, the prevalence of PIMS was 38.8%, consistent with previously published foreign [1–3]. This problem occurs more often in the first 3 months of life and increases the risk of supplementation by 3.4 times. Overall, the negative impact of PIMS is associated with a significant reduction in the average duration of EBF (by 1 month) and BF (by 4 months).

A number of predictors of PIMS had statistically significant different frequencies in the groups, but were not included in the multifactorial model. The analysis showed that mothers with no BF experience (first pregnancy and childbirth) were more likely to experience PIMS. Along with this, cesarean delivery is a negative predictor for lactation initiation, which is explained by disrupted physiological processes of transition from lactogenesis I to lactogenesis II and further to lactogenesis III. The presence of a more educated father in the family contributes to successful lactation, but the mother's education as a separate predictor is irrelevant to this.

At the maternity hospital stage, separation of mother and child, sex of the newborn, and gestational age had no effect on the risk of PIMS at an older age. The woman's desire to breastfeed, the parents' age, and the family's financial status were also irrelevant to the formation of this problem. All these factors occurred with equal frequency in the compared groups and were not included in the multifactorial model.

The dynamics of weight gain in infants were more often statistically significantly different between the groups, but these differences were not clinically significant. All indicators were within the range recommended by WHO and national guidelines. It was not possible to calculate a multifactorial model of the effect of anthropometric parameters on the risk of PIMS.

In this study, eight predictors had the main influence on the risk of PIMS. Construction of a multivariate logistic regression model allowed to estimate the significance of the influence of each of eight predictors on the risk of PIMS. The influence of all factors was quite logically related to each other. For example, late first latch (p_5) requires the introduction of formula into the baby's diet in the maternity hospital (p_4). This disrupts the physiological establishment of lactation, which after discharge from the maternity hospital requires the continuation of supplementation with formula feedings (p_1) to the baby and regular expressions (p_2) for an adequate nutritional status of the baby. Separating the mother and baby in the first half of the year (p_3) with formula feeding and introducing additional fluids (p_7) to the infant only aggravate the situation—the risk of PIMS increases significantly. The mother's education level (p_8) has no protective effect in this situation. Lack of prenatal preparation for breastfeeding (p_6) worsens the prognosis for successful lactation.

4. Conclusion

Thus, our study identified eight main predictors that increase the risk of PIMS in breastfeeding mothers, which in turn reduces the duration of EBF and BF. To reduce the risk of PIMS, pregnant women should receive good prenatal education, follow WHO recommendations strictly in the maternity hospital (early first latch, avoid introducing of formula to healthy children in the maternity hospital and after discharge) and after discharge (mother and healthy baby sleep together, elimination of unnecessary expressions, elimination of introduction of additional liquid to the breast milk) are necessary.

Author details

Yakov Y. Yakovlev
Novokuznetsk State Institute for Further Training of Physicians – Branch Campus of the Federal State Budgetary Educational Institution of Further Professional Education "Russian Medical Academy of Continuous Professional Education" of the Ministry of Healthcare of the Russian Federation

*Address all correspondence to: yko3@yandex.ru

References

[1] Wambach K. In: Wambach K, Spencer B, editors. Breastfeeding and Human Lactation. 6th ed. Burlington, Massachusetts: Jones & Bartlett Learning; 2019. p. 820

[2] Lawrence RA. In: Lawrence RA, Lawrence RM, Noble L, Rosen-Carole C, Stuebe AM, editors. Breastfeeding: A Guide for the Medical Profession. Philadelphia, PA: Elsevier; 2022. p. 1088

[3] Gatti L. Maternal perceptions of insufficient milk supply in breastfeeding. Journal of Nursing Scholarship: An Official Publication of Sigma Theta Tau International Honor Society of Nursing. 2008;**40**(4):355-363. DOI: 10.1111/j.1547-5069.2008.00234.x

[4] Hill PD. Insufficient milk supply. Image—The Journal of Nursing Scholarship. 1989;**21**(3):145-148

[5] World Health Organization. Infant and Young Child Feeding Counselling: An Integrated Course: Participant's Manual. Geneva, Switzerland: U.N.C. Fund (UNICEF)—World Health Organization; 2021. p. xiii, 603

Chapter 8

Breastfeeding Multiples

Jennifer Ayton and Emily Hansen

Abstract

How do women experience breastfeeding multiples? Given the rising rate of multiple births and the global public health target of increasing the number of women exclusively breastfeeding up to the first 6 months, it is imperative that we understand why women who give birth to multiple babies breastfeed for shorter durations compared to those who have one baby. This chapter will explore the qualitative experiences of mothers who breastfeed twins/triplets and the social and physical capital women use to support multiple breastfeeding. Paying close attention to the mothers' personal accounts this chapter will detail the many resources women draw on to meet the challenges of breastfeeding twins and triplets.

Keywords: breastfeeding, mothers, twin, triplets, qualitative, capital, Bourdieu

1. Introduction

1.1 Breastfeeding

Substantial evidence exists to support the global public health recommendation of exclusive breastfeeding, meaning feeding young infants only breast milk for the first 6 months of life, whether directly from the breast or expressed (including milk from donors) [1, 2]. Short and long-term health benefits of exclusive and continued breastfeeding for up to 1–2 years of life in all contexts are well documented. These include reduced risk of breast and ovarian cancer, immunological protection for the infant against infections (including diarrheal, respiratory tract, and ear), no growth faltering, reduced incidence of diabetes and obesity in later life, and increased intelligence [2–5].

In high-income countries, a strong protective effect was found against sudden infant death syndrome (reduced risk of 36%)—and against infant and childhood infections, (diarrheal and respiratory tract), and dental malocclusions. There was also a reduced risk of childhood and adult obesity and diabetes and increases in intelligence. No relationship was found for allergic conditions (such as asthma) or cardiovascular-related diseases, including hypertension. The authors found an increase in tooth decay in children who breastfed nocturnally for longer periods, beyond 12 months of age. Across all settings, exclusive breastfeeding offered protection against life-threatening diseases such as gastroenteritis, and to a lesser extent respiratory infections [2]. The benefits are age and dose respondent; with extended exclusivity increasing protection into the second year of life. Combined observational and clinical trials provide strong evidence to support continued exclusive breastfeeding for up to 6 months, showing that the delayed feeding of non-breast milk fluids (formula milk, water, teas, and juice) or foods did not cause any faltering in infant growth or nutritional compromise for infants in their first year of life [6, 7]. Despite the numerous health, economic, and social benefits.

1.2 Patterns of exclusive breastfeeding

The WHO and UNICEF 2015's Fifth Global Nutrition Target is to increase the rate of exclusive breastfeeding in the first 6 months by up to 50% [1]. This aligns with and supports the United Nations Sustainable Development Goals numbers 2—No hunger, 3—Good health and well-being, and 10-reduced inequalities [8]. Increasing exclusive breastfeeding could prevent 823,000 annual deaths in children younger than 5 years and 20,000 annual deaths from breast cancer [2].

Breastfeeding practices are highly variable across countries and settings. In low and middle-income countries rates of initiation within the first 24 hours range from 80 to 50% with a global weighted prevalence of 51.9%. In many well-resourced countries such as the United Kingdom and Australia, initiation rates are between 70 and 90% and the proportion of infants exclusively breastfeeding to 6 months is lower (2–35%) [9, 10] compared to low and middle-income settings, with the weighted prevalence of 45.7% 2010–2018 [11–13].

Indeed, there has been a noticeable downward trend in exclusive breastfeeding across the globe. It is estimated that two out of three infants worldwide are not exclusively breastfed [14] and only 32–37% of infants are exclusively breastfed worldwide [2].

Data from the first National Infant Feeding survey in Australia, in 2010 showed an initiation rate of 96%, noting a steady decline in exclusivity within the first 4 months after birth (39%) and any breastfeeding for each month of age after that [10]. The most recent data (2021) from Australia estimates that one in three (35.4%) of infants are exclusively breastfed to 6 months of age [9]. These rates fall dramatically short of global targets of 50% of infants exclusively breastfeeding feeding at 6 months [12, 15].

1.3 Breastfeeding twins and triplets

In 2020, multiple pregnancies (birth of two or mother infants) represented 1.5% of all births in Australia and have risen in other high-income counties. About 98% of multiple births are twins. Only 2% were "other multiples" such as triplets, quadruplets or higher. The proportion of multiple births is higher among older mothers, aged >40 years and lowest for young and teenage mothers aged <20 years (0.8%). These patterns are thought to be associated with an increase in the use of assisted reproductive technology (ART) for women aged >36 years [16, 17].

Multiple births are not without adverse risks for the mother and infant. It is estimated that there is a 50% increased risk of preterm birth (a baby born <37 completed weeks gestation), low birth weight (born <2500 g), congenital malformations and infant mortality. For the mother, they are more likely to have a caesarean section, delayed initiation of breastfeeding, mother-infant separation, lack of skin-to-skin, longer hospital admission and delayed recovery time [16].

Consequently, multiple births increase the challenges mothers and their partners face when choosing to breastfeed. Breastfeeding rates (initiation and exclusive) are lower for multiples compared to a singleton. Mothers of multiples are less likely to choose to breastfeed, initiate and offer any breastfeeding [10]. Physical factors such as prematurity, and low birth weight, predispose the infant to developmental and physiological immaturity- contributing to poor temperature regulation and lengthy hospital stays in neonatal intensive care units, the inability to feed at the breast due to immature feeding reflexes. All these factors contribute to delays in initiation, demand for the mother to express breastmilk over lengthy periods, poor milk supply, mother-infant separation, maternal anxiety, and poor breastfeeding outcomes [18–20].

Research about breastfeeding has focused on the duration of exclusive and breastfeeding for singleton infants, and little attention has been given to the experiences of mothers who give birth to multiple babies. This study undertook a secondary analysis of qualitative data to explore the experiences of mothers who were feeding twins/triplets and how they navigated multiple breastfeeding.

2. Theoretical frameworks

An important theoretical concept guiding the analysis of the findings in this study is the concept of capital as outlined by the French Sociologist, Pierre Bourdieu. Bourdieu's definition of *capital* includes three types economic (i.e., money), social (family, social groups) and cultural/symbolic (i.e., education) [21]. The value of capital is realised when other types of capital are exchanged to benefit the individual in their social context. For example, Bourdieu viewed the body as a type of biological and social "physical capital" used to gain social status and cultural capital in the form of higher educational attainment may be used to gain employment, and money [22].

3. The study

This study was conducted in Tasmania, Australia, a southern Island state with a population of 558,00, 2022. Approximately, 6000 women gave birth in 2015 when the study was first conducted, compared to 5,560,2020–1.8% of the total number of women who gave birth in Australia (291,710) [23]. The number of women giving birth in Tasmania, and therefore making decisions about how to feed their newborns has decreased over a 5-year period. Approximately 1.4% of those were multiple (twins/triplets) births. The proportion of mothers giving birth to twins/triplets is slightly higher in Tasmania, at 1.5% [23].

The Tasmanian Infant Feeding Study (TIF) was a mixed methods study that involved 127 mothers and their infants aged from 0 through to 36 months, conducted in 2015. The aim of the study was to explore how mothers spoke about their infant feeding practices and experiences. This mixed methods study consisted of multiple forms of qualitative data (focus groups and semi-structured interviews) researcher field notes recorded after focus groups and interviews and quantitative data from a short survey collecting information about mother and infant demographic and health-related information and feeding practices. Participants (mothers) completed a mother and infant demographic and infant feeding practices questionnaire prior to participating in either a semi-structured FG (22 focus groups were held) and/or a semi-structured interview (19 interviews were conducted) reported elsewhere [28]. Of the 127 mothers who participated in the study, 6 had given birth to twins and 1 to triplets.

This current study consisted of secondary analysis of multiple forms of qualitative data, focus groups, interviews, researcher field notes and some quantitative demographic survey data. Mixed methods have been heavily used within social sciences and public health research. It is common practice to rely on one of the methods (e.g., qualitative) to provide deeper insights into the specific phenomenon [24]. In this study integration of both quantitative demographic and qualitative data occurred at the point of data analysis and interpretation. The mothers' demographics were linked to the transcripts using the soft wear package NVivo through the unique demographic questionnaire identification number and pseudonyms. This facilitated cross-checking of participants' characteristics with emerging themes, sources, references, and ensured adequate participant representation and across and within the analytic categories [24].

3.1 Sampling

In the original study a purposeful sampling was used to include a range of information-rich cases [25]. Mothers were recruited from rural and urban areas of Tasmania. The inclusion criteria included: mothers 16 years and over with infants aged between 0 and 36 months. Mothers did not have to be breastfeeding at the time of the data collection to support infant feeding to be explored in a wider context of women's everyday lives. Recruitment strategies included sampling from pre-existing mothers/parenting support groups, mothers, and health professionals, snowball sampling, advertising, and promoting the study within newspapers and posters at community clinics and hospitals.

For the secondary analysis purposeful sampling was used to identify women who had reported through the survey that they had given birth to twins or triplets.

3.2 Data collection and analysis

Mother and infant characteristics (age, highest educational attainment, employment, status, marital status, parity, singleton, multiple births, and postcode) and their current feeding practices were collected prior to the start of each interview and FG using a demographic questionnaire.

Participants could elect to participate in an interview or FG. All FGs (22) and interviews (19) were undertaken in the community setting at convenient times for the mothers and were either naturally occurring or constructed. Two members of the research team gathered the qualitative data using a question guide. Interviews were conducted in person with one researcher in the mother's home. Survey and qualitative data were linked through a unique participant ID number. For the secondary analysis, de-identified data (demographic and interview/FG transcripts) were extracted from the main data base using this ID and imported into a separated password protected data base.

3.3 Data analysis

This paper reports a secondary thematic analysis of data from the seven mothers who gave birth to multiples and of other mothers (n = 2 interviews and 4 FGs) where participants spoke with each other about infant feeding in relation to friends and family experiences. These conversations mainly took place in the FGs. Just over a quarter of the participants (N = 127) had referred to family or friends who had experienced multiple birth and feeding. This data was sought using text searches using the "query" option within NVivo to verify the frequency of use and relevance of key concepts [26] For example, all transcripts were searched for the terms *twin, multiple, triplet, babies*, this helped to identify and explain how mothers talked about their friends and family. Stata/SE 17.0 was used to descriptively analyse demographic data.

Preliminary data analysis allowed for a broad coding framework to be developed. Preliminary codes included: breastfeeding best for baby, care and helpers, multiple mumming, and "other" feeding. These were then thematically reduced into one large thematically driven parent node: capital. Thematically reducing the data using Bourdieu's concept of capital was achieved by selecting and abstracting, sorting and isolating patterns and relationships between variables, and finding commonalities and differences to support formalizing the emerging themes [27]. The node "capital" (and all references and sources) was expanded and reduced theoretically into two principal parent nodes (*physical and social capital*) with relevant sub-nodes. The final theme "Allofeeding" refers to the multiple resources (capital) mothers used to negotiate feeding multiple babies.

4. Findings

In this section pseudonyms and age are used to provide context. We begin by describing the mothers' characteristics analysis. This is followed by an interpretation and discussion of Capital and Allofeeding and related sub-themes using the findings of the analysis.

4.1 Who participated in the study?

Mothers in the TIF study were from a broad demographic and are reported elsewhere [28]. For those who had multiple births and were included in this analysis (N = 7) the mean age was 30.4 years (two mothers were aged <24 years), the highest education level achieved was a graduate diploma for five and three reported home duties/unemployed as occupation, with the reminder professional or sales/service. Four reported being married/living in with a partner, and three were single parents at the time of the study.

At the time of the study infants were > 12 months of age, mean age of 18 months. Three-quarters (5) of the infants were born <2500 g, and premature <37 completed weeks gestation. Only one mother had intended to mix feed (formula and breastmilk), with six intending to breastfeed after birth. None of the women were exclusively breastfeeding at the time of the study, two were mixed feeding (breastmilk and formula).

4.2 Capital

Bourdieu's concept of *capital* can be employed to explore how mothers exchange their physical and social resources during their struggle to breastfeed their twins or triplets. Bourdieu referred to three principal types of capital (economic, social and cultural): in the context of breastfeeding this included economic capital available for consumption/purchase such as money, formula milk, bottles, teats, feeding/shrouds blankets, pillows and sourcing advice via private consults with relevant health care practitioners cultural capital in the form of bodily characteristics and functions, education levels, knowledge, breastmilk, and social capital such as family, friends, fathers and relevant health professionals accessed via social networks [29].

The exchange of capital may occur in either a positive or negative way, generating additional resources or limiting the use of others. Duplication and mutations exist. For example, in this study, using breast milk—either expressed or directly feeding from the breasts—is exchanged for personal, social, and health profits (such as 'good mothering, self-esteem, the health of the baby) [21].

Capital in its symbolic (generating status) or material forms (money, education, breast milk) represents objective and subjective resources [29], that are available to the mother during her time mothering twins/triplets. For example, a mother's physical ability to lactate (produce milk) and choice to breastfeed are embodied as physical capital and provide know how. In the following quote, Sally (26) talks about her body as a resource to feed her triplets:

> *they were born at 32 weeks by caesarean. Luke was in NICU, so he was being drip feed and had a gastric tube and the girls could breathe, but they were being tube feed. I was expressing colostrum like when you start and I found that really easy. It was like my body knew I had triplets and it was just producing huge amounts of colostrum. So that wasn't a problem, but they were being supplemented with formula through the tubes. They couldn't breastfeed because they were too small. It probably took the girls two weeks before they'd start to breastfeed and Luke much longer because he was small. So I was expressing and I reckon I got up to expressing two litres of breast milk a day. It was huge amounts. (Sally)*

This conscious and unconscious know how appears to come from both the acknowledgment of bodily physical capital [21], such as lactating breasts and experiences shared in the family cycle or peer social cycles.

4.3 Allofeeding

This thematic category uses the concept of capital to explore the practice of *allofeeding*. Allofeeding refers to "other-feeding" resources (forms of physical or material capital) that mothers spoke about and use to negotiate caring for and feeding their babies. Allofeeding does not replace the mother but facilitates and supports her in feeding her infant. It is essentially where the mother exchanges her body's physical capital (milk and breasts) and hands over her role as the physical feeder to another.

Allofeeding is therefore a form of capital exchange (breasts, milk, nipples, fathers, kin), that mothers have available as they navigate to feed. In this study, these fell into two groups, social (others) and physical forms of capital (breasts, bottles, other milk). Allofeeding, like the broader concept of allomothering means the shared care of the young infant. Anthropologist Blaffer Hrdy (2009), describes allomothering as:

> *They [infants] have available to them [the mothers'] entire social world. The mother is the principal caretaker ... suckling is frequent and often but by no means always on demand. Without allomothering we would not have a human race [30], p. 75–76*

For mothers who were breastfeeding multiples, allofeeding methods included bottles, teats, milk, their bodies, experts- such as lactation consultants, lay support organisations, and fathers, family, and friends. Allofeeding supports the exchange of "capital" offering the primary feeder support during the process of intensive feeding [21]. In the context of multiple mothering/feeding the mother proffers the role of the primary feeder [30] and thus exchanges her physical capital (breasts and milk) for another form of capital, such as expressing breast milk.

Women in this study employed multiple types of allofeeding to negotiate the breastfeeding of their twins and triplets. The women's accounts of what helped them feed their babies included the use of fathers/partners, and to a lesser degree "kin"—sisters, grandmothers and female friends or other mothers. Second to these were consumable tools such as expressing equipment, dummies, bottles, and teats, expressing equipment. Mothers felt that these resources were "essential" for them to manage the day-to-day feeding of multiple babies.

4.4 Exchange of social and physical capital

Mothers were productive in their use of allofeeding, tailoring the use of commercial products such as bottles, dummies, teats, and formula as resources to suit their unique situation. Bottles, teats, and formula milk are consumer capital. As commodities they were a way to "keep sane," to give the mother a break and allow significant others to feed the babies. As a form of capital -these feeding tools, were converted into emotional and physical support. In the following quote, Alex (24) describes her desire to breastfeed and how she used bottles and formula to give her the commodity of time,

> *I want to try and give it a go breastfeeding, because it's just like easier. Especially because I had the twins, just the bottles was were a nightmare. But whatever I can do. If I can do it, I can do it. See how it goes. It might be a bit easier just to bottle feed this time, because I've got the twins so I'm a bit flat out, so it will be just easier to make up formula. Instead of sitting down for two or three hours at a time trying to feed a baby, and then get up and do all the of it again...that's what they [health professionals] need to understand too, that mums like us have extra children, we don't have the time. Because bottle feeding can go much faster. When you've got other children you don't have the time to spend with them, and it does, it takes ages. (Alex, 24)*

The emotional and physical demands of breastfeeding multiple babies, as Samantha (28) said, being "the only one who can feed" and producing "enough milk" placed a great deal of strain on these mothers. They often spoke about what they perceived as their lack of freedom when breastfeeding, and the importance of being able to gain some respite from the constant demands of feeding:

> *Yeah, I'm just exhausted I'm with them [twins] 24/7. (Alex 24)*

> *Yeah, my friend had triplets and it [trying to breastfeed] nearly tipped her over the edge. (Samantha, 28)*

> *Wow ... couldn't do that (Petra, 30)*

The feeling of exhaustion does not reflect the mothers' deep personal desire to breastfeed [28]. Indeed, all seven women described the importance of providing breast milk either through expressing breast milk or feeding directly from the breast. However, there was a palpable need among the mothers to share the role so that they could continue breastfeeding. This often generated a feeling of conflict because of the desire "do it all" and "do what is right" and the need to "share the load" (Rose, 35). As the quote below suggests, this tension was heightened for mothers with twins as they talked about the demands of multiple mothering.

> *I think it also takes a lot of energy to breastfeed twins, and you need to try and eat properly, and it also takes time ..you spend a lot of time on the couch. But if you've just given birth, you're on the couch anyway...too much milk or too much supply, your boobs start to get really sore...there's too much of everything. (Petra, 30)*

Mothers expected themselves—and perceived that they were expected by others—to breastfeed because "it is natural." This reification of 'natural' symbolises the ideology of a "good mother," a mother who sacrifices her body (physical capital) to meet the needs of her dependent infant [31]. However, for the mothers with twins/triplets, the message they received was to "lower their expectations" because it [breastfeeding] was not going to be as they expected. For this reason, women with multiples appeared to pragmatically accept the need for other commercial resources, bottles, teats, dummies and expressing equipment. These tools were all part of their role as the mother of multiples. The use of this type of commercial capital offered them opportunities to share their bodily capital, in exchange for a break, in exchange for a break as Rose describes below:

> *...with breastfeeding that was something that was important to me, and knowing that I am doing the best thing for my babies. But also with bottle feeding, whether it was expressed milk or whether now it's cow's milk, I think it's nice for my husband to be able to bottle feed as well, so he can share the cuddling and that nice time, and I can sleep. (Rose, 35)*

Converting their bodily physical capital (breasts and milk) and mobilising others such as fathers and others (social capital) to provide relief and support through bottle feeding was a consistent issue raised by other women feeding twins/triplets in the study:

> *I wanted to sleep, probably still wanted to sleep. So I'd twin feed two of them. I had a great breastfeeding pillow that you can't buy in the shops. It was made by a twin mum. So you could sit that on the couch around you and the two could twin feed and I could put a dinner plate in the middle and eat. I was constantly eating. So it never had that beautiful bonding breastfeeding that other people talk about and I'd either have my nanny or my husband for every feed giving a bottle to the third one and it would rotate. We'd have a roster up so that they all got equal amounts of breastfeeding and bottle feeding. (Rebecca, 31)*

The physical and emotional demands of simultaneously breastfeeding multiple infants were also experienced by women who bottle-fed (with breast milk or formula) while breastfeeding, in addition to those who exclusively bottle-fed using expressed breastmilk and formula milk. For these women, the advantage of bottles was that they could physically hand over (exchange) the baby and the feeding to another for the reward of returning to work, social outings:

> *So the formula was introduced for the six pm and that gave me a bit of a break. We'd give the kids the six pm bottle and all the adults would have a glass of wine, that was the ritual. That was a lovely time, bottles and alcohol for everyone and then I stopped expressing, so they used up what was in the freezer and then they went to the formula for the third one and it's hard to remember now. When I was cutting it all out, I went back to just breastfeeding one of them... because I was worried about her allergies and then that's how I cut it down. Cutting down was really easy. I thought it would be hard, but it wasn't. Yeah, but what did it was me saying to my husband I can't cope and he said you have to and I thought okay well what do I do. All I can do is give up breastfeeding, so that's what I had to do. It was the only option left. (Deb, 30)*
>
> *Q. And you felt relief once you did?*

A. Oh totally, yeah. Wish I'd done it sooner. I wish I'd had the bonding.

For mothers with twins/triplets using multiple forms of capital (social and physical) such as getting someone else to help feed the baby was the great benefit of using bottles. Conversely, Samantha (28), who had four children including twins, described a sense of guilt because she could not meet the demands of multiple breastfeeding her twins while also caring for other young children:

Having a double breast pump [laughter from the other mothers] was a real flattering look and caring for four young children and to try to get them on the boob ... ehhh. It was okay when my partner was off work, but as soon as he went back ... I just couldn't manage. (Samantha)

4.5 Pressure

All mothers in the study referred to a feeling of "pressure to breastfeed." They discussed this in relation to their own "high expectations," partners'/husbands' feeding preferences, generic health information about the nutritional benefits of breastmilk and avoidance of bottles, and health professionals' advice. Many of the participants had no frame of reference for feeding and learning to breastfeed multiple babies. They describe how the reality was a shock because they had not been exposed to twin feeding before:

Well I don't know for mums of one baby because I've just got no idea what that pressures like or to bottle feed or not. For me having experience of other twin mum's would have been good. Mum's that said no I didn't breastfeed because the books that they give you is all about the mum's that do twin breastfeed and how you can do it, go girl you can do this. Don't let people pressure you, that you should breastfeed, that you can do it. In the little booklet that they give you, there was nothing that said it's okay to have formula as well as breast milk. So that would have helped now... Some support that that's okay to do both. Don't give it up completely and go to formula. You can still do both. (Rebecca, 31)

For mothers of twins and triplets, the pressure and sense of failure after stopping exclusive breastfeeding appeared mitigated by the increased care burden of multiple babies. Consequently, using formula milk was felt to be an acceptable outcome of a multiple births, as Petra (30) stated "you have twins how can you do it all." Unlike mothers of singleton infants [28], twin/triplet mothers did not appear to struggle with the same depth of guilt and regret about stopping breastfeeding. Their experiences of ceasing to breastfeed were related to the "relentless" demands of caring and the unrecognised strain this placed on their bodies and mental health [19]. As such breastfeeding directly from the breast was the one task that could be traded- exchanged to afford the mother a break and as many women explained some sanity. This often led to a pragmatic decision to use formula milk. In the following quote, Deb (30) describes the relief she felt when she stopped breastfeeding,

The fact that I was doing it [breastfeeding] meant to me that I should keep doing it. What would be the signal to stop? There was no obvious signal because you can't assess your own mental health when you're in it. There was no warning light to say

> *you're falling apart. It was not like my milk dried up or anything. It was just coming and coming and coming.*
>
> *Q. How did you feel when you stopped?*
>
> *A. Relief. I wished id done it sooner. (Deb)*

For Deb, exchanging her embodied capital (breasts and milk) with bottles and formula milk offered her the opportunity to protect her mental health and well-being; another form of capital necessary for her to meet the needs of her family and self.

4.6 Expressing

For Bourdieu capital is most valuable when it is exchanged. Expressing milk and the use of bottles is the result of the exchange of two forms of bodily capital (breast and milk) and commercial capital, the mother's purchase, and use of bottles and/or teats and expressing equipment. All seven mothers expressed breastmilk. Collectively experiencing expressing breastmilk as challenging, and time-consuming. For some mothers, the exchange of their milk and use of bottles and teats was a welcome form of allofeeding. Petra (30) described the practice of expressing for her twins as "gold... yeah, because you feed off one side and then express the other, but I didn't do that –just fed and then expressed if I needed to".

Others talked of expressing and bottle feeding as a loss of autonomy, but a necessity. Alex (24) like other mothers, felt she had little choice but to express breast milk because she was constantly exhausted. She counted herself lucky because of her excess milk supply, stating that she felt "blessed with a huge supply." Many women described how they had to and were advised to "double pump" soon after birth because their babies were too small to feed at the breast, otherwise, they would not "last the distance" and have enough for two babies. Others shared how it made them feel objectified... "like a cow." Sally (26) explained that "it [expressing] wasn't a tasteful thing to do and the expressing machines...quite gross too."

Expressing and using bottles had a role in helping mothers to negotiate the extra care burden of breastfeeding multiple babies. In this context expressing breastmilk is used as a resource that can be exchanged for social and bodily freedoms, allowing mothers to continue to provide some breastmilk, while exchanging breast milk as a product that can be shared and benefit the health of the baby. Moreover, the provision of expressed breastmilk allowed the mother to retain the social status of a good mother, doing the best for her baby and continuing to "do what is right and give them some breast milk" (Samantha, 28).

4.7 Fathers

For coupled mothers' collaborative partnerships with the father of the infant appeared to be beneficial. Mothers described feeling less burdened by the "full-time" demands of breastfeeding twins/triplets when they were able to share some of the care demands with their partners. It was clear that support from the infants' fathers created an opportunity for continued breastfeeding. Rose (30), talked about how sharing the role of feeding with her partner allowed her to work through feeding issues while feeding her twins:

> *...it wasn't so bad when my other half was off work but as soon as he went back to work it was, just had no time all I was doing was pretty much feeding the twins flat out because I was doing one at a time because one wouldn't latch on properly and it just hurt like crazy. (Rose)*

The father's/partners investment in the mother and infants places them in the position of an allofeeder. In the context of multiple births, this role appeared to be separate from other external forms of commercial or social capital as multiple birth support groups, family members, nannies, economic support from government sources, and twin pillows. As in other studies, it was clear that the father of the infant was the most significant form of social capital for the breastfeeding mother with twins/triplets. As Rebecca (31) said, "because he [the father of the infant] was very involved, and I really supported him being involved right from the start." However, for some women who felt pressured to breastfeed the fathers' involvement generated some tension. In the following quote, Sally (26) a mother of triplets shares how the exchange of capital (father's time and investment) can be both positive and negative. Sally gains some symbolic capital (social acceptance and standing) by successfully breastfeeding her triplets – being a "good mother" but this is felt as both a gain and a loss.

> *The breastfeeding was going well, but I felt pressured because it was going well and everyone was telling me what a wonderful job I was doing. But I didn't want to be doing it and I felt guilty because I didn't want to be doing it. But everyone was going oh aren't you great, aren't you wonderful and my husband was bragging to everyone, but deep down I was like oh please I wish I didn't have to do this [breastfeeding]. (Sally, 26)*

Overall, allofeeding, particularly when the father of the baby is involved, appeared to provide some benefits to the mother and father collectively as a care and feeding unit. The mother's partner and her physical capital (breast and milk) appeared to be exchanged as capital for the benefit of the multiple-family unit.

5. Conclusion

In this chapter, we have explored how Bourdieu's concept of capital helps to view the mother's breastfeeding body as a form of physical capital that offers a profitable return for multiple birth families- mother, father/partner, and babies. The return is often increased social status, such as a perception of being a good mother and improving the health of the babies through providing breastmilk. In this secondary analysis of women's experiences of feeding their twins/triplet babies, women used many forms of physical and social capital to help them negotiate the increased care and feeding demands. These included using fathers/partners, bottles, formula milk, expressing equipment and teats and all represent a form of allofeeding.

While the challenges of breastfeeding may be higher for the mothers of multiples the pressure to breastfeed (exclusively or any) appeared to be mitigated by the perceived demands of a multiple births. The use of allofeeding (of bottles, teats, formula milk, and expressing equipment) was accepted and normalised as part of the process of feeding multiple babies. For the twin/triplet mother the need to convert social and physical capital to manage the extra care demands was palpable. The conversion of capital, therefore, supports the mental and emotional well-being of the mother by allowing her to share the care and pressures to breastfeed. In turn, the act of breastfeeding multiples whether through expressed breastmilk and or feeding from the breast generates numerous types of capital for both mother and baby, including symbolic capital—where the mother's body is used to double the social return—reinforcing the social ideology of "good mothering" [31, 32].

Acknowledgements

We would like to acknowledge the funding from the Tasmanian Early Years Association and the contribution of the women who participated in this study.

Conflict of interest

The authors declare no conflict of interest.

Author details

Jennifer Ayton[1*] and Emily Hansen[2]

1 School of Medicine, College of Health and Medicine, University of Tasmania, Hobart, Australia

2 School of Social Sciences, College of Arts Law and Education, University of Tasmania, Hobart, Australia

*Address all correspondence to: jennifer.ayton@utas.edu.au

References

[1] World Health Organisation/UNICEF. Global Nutrition Targets 2025: Breastfeeding Policy Brief. Geneva: World Health Organization (WHO); 2014

[2] Victora CG et al. Breastfeeding in the 21st century: Epidemiology, mechanisms, and lifelong effect. Lancet. 2016;**387**(10017):475-490

[3] Horta BL. Breastfeeding: Investing in the future. Breastfeeding Medicine. 2019;**14**(S1):S-11-S-12

[4] Horta BL, de Lima NP. Breastfeeding and type 2 diabetes: Systematic review and meta-analysis. Current Diabetes Reports. 2019;**19**(1):1-6

[5] Horta BL, Loret de Mola C, Victora CG. Long-term consequences of breastfeeding on cholesterol, obesity, systolic blood pressure and type 2 diabetes: A systematic review and meta-analysis. Acta Paediatrica. 2015;**104**:30-37

[6] Bhutta ZA. Early nutrition and adult outcomes: Pieces of the puzzle. Lancet. 2013;**382**(9891):486-487

[7] Kramer M, Kakuma R. Optimal duration of exclusive breastfeeding (review). Cochrane Database of Systematic Reviews. 2012;**8**:CD003517

[8] SDG U. Sustainable Development Goals. United Nations; 2015

[9] Australian Bureau of Statistics. Breastfeeding: Key Statistics and Data about Breastfeeding, Exclusive Breastfeeding, and Introduction to Solid Foods. National Health Survey: First Results. Canberra, Australia: Australian Bureau of Statistics (ABS). 2022 [cited 2022 October]. Available from: https://www.abs.gov.au/statistics/health/health-conditions-and-risks/breastfeeding/latest-release#methodology

[10] Australian Institute of Health and Welfare. 2010 Australian National Infant Feeding Survey: Indicator Results. Australian Government: Canberra; 2011

[11] World Health Organization. World Health Statistics 2013. Geneva: World Health Organization; 2015

[12] World Health Organization. UNICEF Global Nutrition Targets 2025: Breastfeeding Policy Brief (WHO/NMH/NHD/14.7). Geneva: World Health Organization; 2014

[13] Wu H, Zhao M. Global prevalence of WHO infant feeding practices in 57 LMICs in 2010-2018 and time trends since 2000 for 44 LMICs. EClinicalMedicine. 2021;**100971**(37):1-9. DOI: 10.1016/j.eclinm.2021.100971

[14] World Health Organization. Health Topics: Breastfeeding. 2016 [cited 2016 12 June]. Available from: http://www.who.int/features/factfiles/breastfeeding/en/

[15] Australian Health Ministers' Conference 2009. The Australian National Breastfeeding Strategy 2010-2015. Australian Government Department of Health and Ageing, Editor: Canberra; 2009

[16] Qin J-B et al. Worldwide prevalence of adverse pregnancy outcomes associated with in vitro fertilization/intracytoplasmic sperm injection among multiple births: A systematic review and meta-analysis based on cohort studies. Archives of Gynecology and Obstetrics. 2017;**295**(3):577-597

[17] Murray S, Norman J. Multiple pregnancies following assisted reproductive technologies–a happy consequence or double trouble? In: Seminars in Fetal and Neonatal Medicine. USA: Elsevier; 2014. DOI: 10.1016/j.siny.2014.03.001

[18] Whitford HM et al. Breastfeeding education and support for women with twins or higher order multiples. Cochrane Database of Systematic Reviews. 2017;**2**:1-46. DOI: 10.1002/14651858.CD012003.pub2

[19] Fisher J, Stocky A. Maternal perinatal mental health and multiple births: Implications for practice. Twin Research and Human Genetics. 2003;**6**(6):506-513

[20] Mikami FCF et al. Breastfeeding twins: Factors related to weaning. Journal of Human Lactation. 2018;**34**(4):749-759

[21] Bourdieu P. The Logic of Practice. Cambridge: Polity; 1990

[22] Robbins D. Pierre Bourdieu. Vol. 1. London: SAGE; 2000

[23] Australian Bureau of Statistics., Snapshot of Tasmania: High level summary data for Tasmania in. 2021. Australia: Australian Bureau of Statistics; 2021

[24] Tashakkori A, Teddlie C. Sage Handbook of Mixed Methods in Social & Behavioral Research. 2nd ed. Los Angeles: SAGE Publications. xv; 2010. p. 893

[25] Creswell JW, Planto Clark VL. Designing and Conducting Mixed Methods Research. 2nd ed. California: SAGE; 2011

[26] Bazeley P, Jackson K. Qualitative Data Analysis with NVivo. London: Sage Publications Limited; 2013

[27] Denzin N, Lincoln Y, editors. The SAGE Handbook of Qualitative Research Fifth Ed. United States Of America: SAGE; 2018

[28] Ayton J, Tesch L, Hansen E. Women's experiences of ceasing to breastfeed: Australian qualitative study. BMJ Open. 2019;**9**(5):e026234

[29] Bourdieu P. Distinction. London: Routledge and Kegan Paul; 1984

[30] Blaffer Hrdy S. Mothers and Others: The Evolutionary Origins of Mutual Understanding 2009. London: Belknap Press of Harvard University Press. 2009

[31] Blum L. At the Breast: Ideologies of Breastfeeding and Motherhood in the Contemporary United States. USA: Beacon Press; 2000

[32] Blum L. Twenty first century virtual mothers or rounded mothers? In: At the Breast: Ideologies of Breastfeeding and Motherhood in the Contemporary United States. Beacon Press: Boston; 2000. pp. 180-201

Section 4

Complication

Chapter 9

Complications of Multiple Pregnancy: Conception to Delivery

Tshililo Mashamba

Abstract

Multiple pregnancy is a condition where more than one fetus occupy the same intrauterine cavity. By means of its rarity in spontaneous pregnancies, it indicates that that by nature the human female uterus is programmed to carry one fetus at a time. The incidence of multiple pregnancy is on the increase because of fertility treatment especially assisted reproductive technology. Unfortunately, multiple pregnancy is associated with several complications from conception until the postpartum period. Maternal uterine anomalies also pose special challenges if associated with multiple pregnancy from diagnosis until management. Miscarriages are higher and some of them are not noticed if the pregnancy continues with one fetus. There are complications related to uterine space like preterm labour which is the commonest. Rupture of membranes with or without preterm labour is also common. Monochorionic multiple pregnancies poses specific challenges in respect to abnormalities during organogenesis from embryonal to vascular malformations. Fetus growth discordance and single twin demise are uncommon but challenging.

Keywords: multiple pregnancy, miscarriages, dichorionic, monochorionic, preterm labour, anomalies, complications

1. Introduction

Multiple pregnancy refers to simultaneous development of more than one fetus in a female. Simultaneous development of two foetuses is called twins and that of three is triplets and four is quadruplets and so on. The incidence of multiple pregnancy 1 about 1% indicating that by nature, human reproduction is programmed to carry and nurture one fetus at a time [1]. The incidence of spontaneous twin pregnancy is 1:90, the incidence of triplets is 1:8000 and the incidence of quadruplets is 1:700000. Among the quadruplets the most frequent is the tetrachorionic tetra-amniotic type. These rates have increased 300–400% due to the development of assisted reproductive techniques. The expected average gestational age at delivery for twins is 36–37 weeks, while for triplets is 33–34 weeks and 30–31 weeks for quadruplets [2]. Multiple pregnancy is associated with several maternal and neonatal complications which will be discussed in this chapter.

IntechOpen

2. Early pregnancy complications

A pregnancy is defined by detection of a positive serum hCG. Biochemical pregnancy is when serum hCG is positive without a detectable gestational sac. The incidence of miscarriages is based on pregnancies where a gestational sac has been detected and report are based on pregnancies following assisted reproduction. Unlike ectopic pregnancies which present with symptoms and their incidence is more reliable. The incidence of miscarriages is estimated to between 12 and 15% of all pregnancies. The number of miscarriages may be two to four fold if early unrecognised miscarriages are included [3]. As many as 60% of all conceptions abort in the first trimester and at least 50% of all losses happened unnoticed [3]. In spontaneous conception, spontaneous miscarriage is more common in multiple pregnancy. It has been suggested that more twins are conceived than born. Three times more twin were observed among aborted pregnancies [4, 5]. The patients who achieve a positive pregnancy test with more than one gestational sac initially are more likely to deliver at least one baby [3]. Therefore, there are patients who were pregnant with more than one fetus who end experience a miscarriage of other fetus(es) being unnoticed. The presence of intrauterine haematoma in the first trimester is associated with the loss of one or both foetuses before 20 weeks of gestation, but the size of the haematoma is not an independent factor [6].

A larger proportion of monozygotic multiple pregnancy were thought to have more genetic aberrations compared to dizygotic embryos and singletons. Contrary to expectation the risk of Downs' syndrome per fetus is lower in multiple pregnancy than in singleton pregnancies. The prevalence of twins with Downs syndrome was lower in with particularly low prevalence in same sex twins [7, 8]. Unlike chromosomal aberrations, structural anomalies have been found to occur more often in monozygotic twins compared with dizygotic twins and singletons. Congenital anomalies may be the results of the teratogenic insult that causes the twinning [9]. The risk of congenital anomalies in monochorionic twins is twice as high compared to dichorionic twins and singletons [10]. Monozygotic twinning itself can be regarded as an abnormality of morphogenesis [11]. The risk of congenital anomalies in twins is higher than in singleton supporting the notion of monozygotic twinning regarded as an morphogenetic anomaly. The anomalies vary from nervous system, cardiovascular, genitourinary and twin specific anomalies like twin reversed arterial perfusion [10].

In early pregnancy there are complications specific for unusual multiple pregnancies types. Heterotopic pregnancy (**Figure 1**) is a rare clinical condition in which intrauterine and extra-uterine pregnancies occur at the same time. The incidence is estimated to be about 1 in 30,000 spontaneous pregnancies while a higher prevalence may occur in assisted reproduction techniques that may reach up to 1 case per 100 in some literatures. It is a challenge to diagnose such a problem due to complex clinical and laboratory findings [12, 13]. Commonly the ectopic pregnancy is within the fallopian tube and uncommonly in the cervix or ovary. Though heterotopic pregnancy is more common following assisted reproduction, cases following spontaneous pregnancies have been reported [14].

The complications expected are a combination if what is expected from an intrauterine pregnancy like abortion and rupture of the fallopian tube from the ectopic pregnancy.

The other unusual type of multiple pregnancy is twin ectopic pregnancy which may be bilateral or unilateral. The incidence of twin ectopic pregnancies (**Figure 2**)

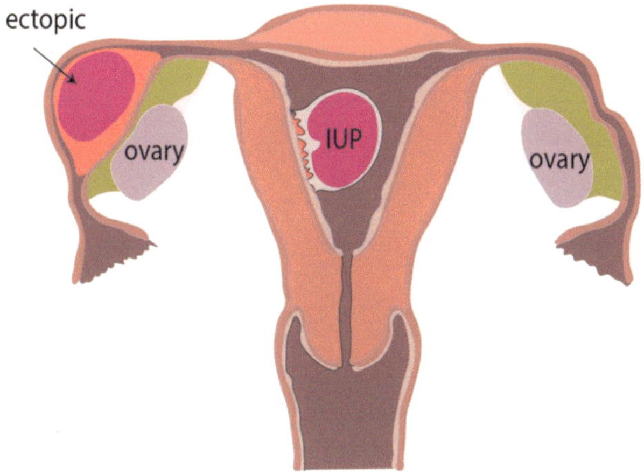

Figure 1.
Heterotopic pregnancy.

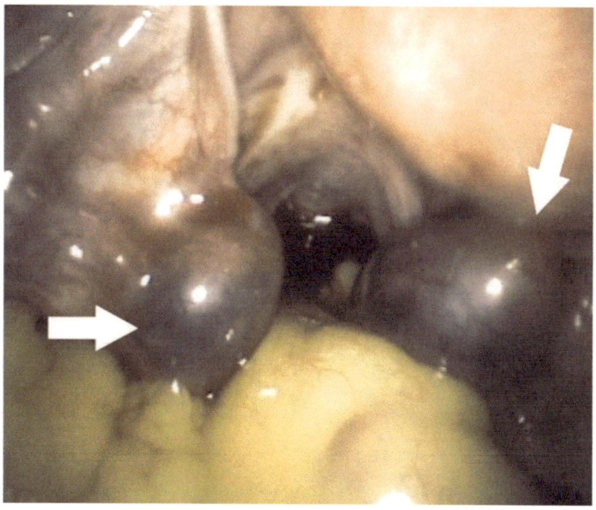

Figure 2.
Bilateral twin ectopic.

is quite rare and is estimated to be 1 in 125,000 pregnancies and 1 in 200 pregnancies following tubal ligation. Many factors increase the risk of ectopic pregnancy, important being pelvic inflammatory disease, pervious pelvic surgery leading to adhesions and assisted reproductive techniques [15]. If not managed timely this can lead to critical complications of severe haemorrhagic shock [16]. The unilateral twin ectopic pregnancy (**Figures 3** and **4**) would appear large due to the presence of two gestational sacs, but gestational age and the corresponding trophoblastic invasion would be less, as compared with a singleton ectopic pregnancy of the same gestational age [17]. Unfortunately, this may not be recognised leading to underestimating the prevalence.

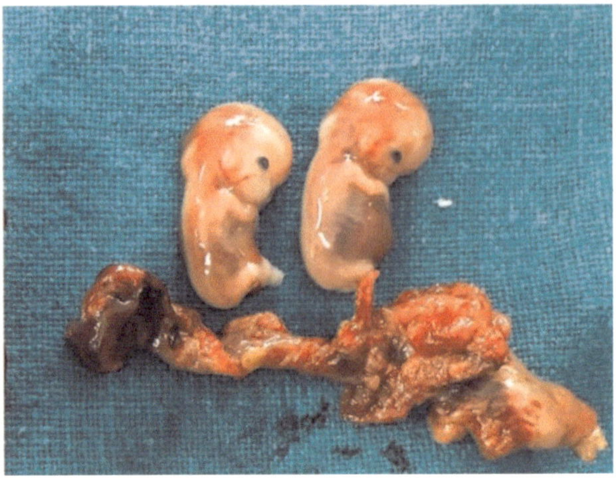

Figure 3.
Ruptured twin ectopic.

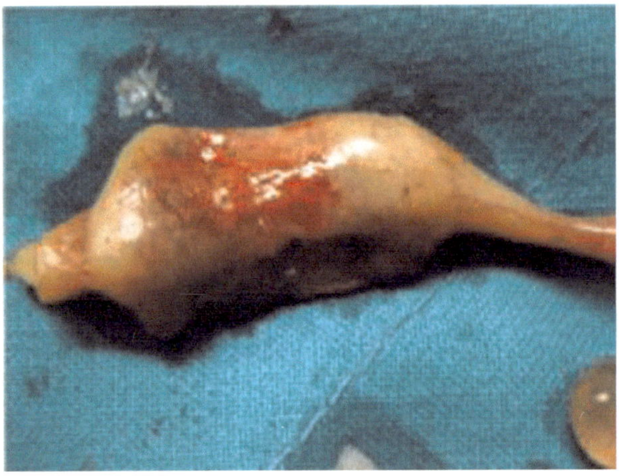

Figure 4.
Unilateral ruptured twin ectopic.

3. Late pregnancy complications

3.1 Preterm labour

Preterm labour is a common complication of multiple pregnancy. This is thought to be secondary to accommodation challenges as the uterus is developed to accommodate one fetus. As this occurs in some patients and not others, the theory may not be completely correct. Elasticity of the uterine muscles should be playing a role on the duration of pregnancy. The prevalence of preterm delivery is higher in patients with uterine anomalies especially with unicornuate [18] or uterine didelphys and is expected to even higher if there is more than one fetus in these anomalies. The other obstetric complications with uterine anomalies are spontaneous miscarriages, preterm delivery, preterm rupture of membranes, intrauterine growth restriction, rudimentary horn rupture and increased need for operative delivery [19]. Congenital uterine anomalies are seen in 1–10% of the general population and are as a result of abnormal formation, fusion or reabsorption of the Mullerian duct. A unicornuate uterus is present in 0.1% of the general population in which an underdeveloped or rudimentary horn may be present (**Figure 5**). Rudimentary horn rupture occurs in 50–90% of cases if the pregnancy is located in this horn [20]. The incidence of rudimentary horn pregnancy as singleton is estimated to be 1 in 76,000–150,000 pregnancies [21] and such pregnancies associated with twins is unknown.

Didelphys uterus correspond to the class III of Mullerian anomalies from the 1988 American Fertility Society classification. Prevalence of all types of female congenital reproductive tract anomalies is estimated at 4–7% and are mostly benign. Uterine didelphys is a rare type of anomaly with estimated prevalence of 0.3%, caused by failure of fusion of the inferior parts of the paramesonephric ducts resulting in separate uterine cavities with 2 cervices and a double or single vagina (**Figures 6** and 7). Uterine didelphys with dicavitary (**Figure 8**) twin pregnancy is exceedingly rare; the reported incidence is 1 in 1,000,000 pregnancies [22, 23]. The complications in uterine didelphys is similar to ones in unicornuate uterus as they are related to accommodation restriction. Such twins are always binovular, the ova being from one or both ovaries. Preterm labour may occur at the same time but unilateral preterm labour has been reported [24].

3.2 Medical conditions associated with multiple pregnancy

1. Anaemia

2. Hypertensive disorders

3. Gestational Diabetes mellitus

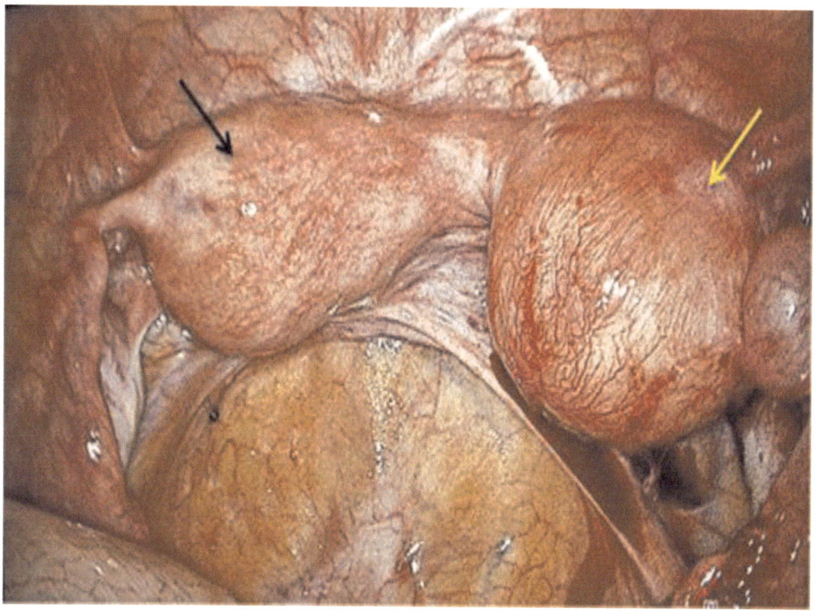

Figure 5.
Unicornuate uterus (black arrow points rudimentary horn and the yellow arrow points to the unicornuate uterus).

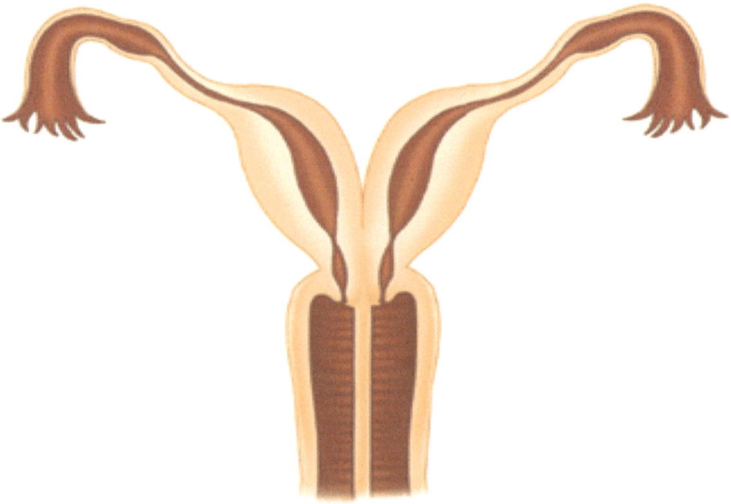

Figure 6.
Didelphys uterus with separate vagina.

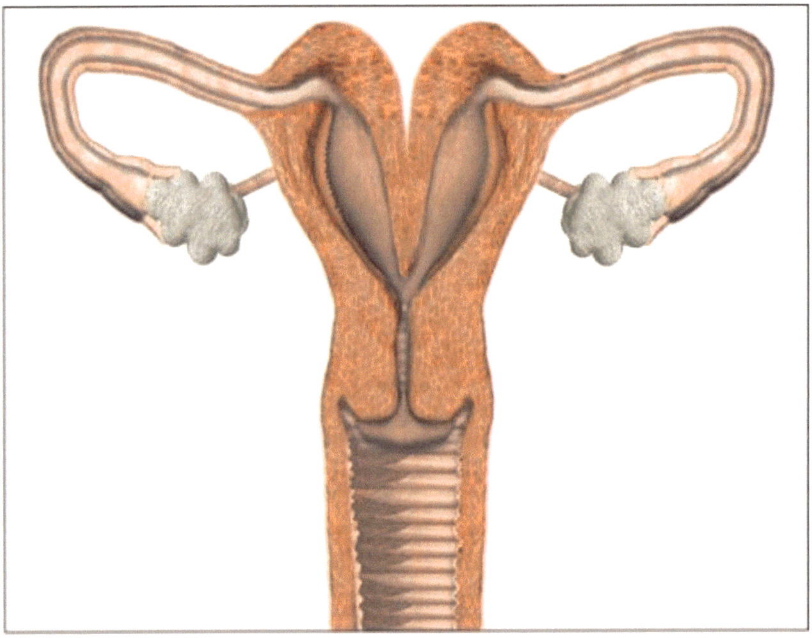

Figure 7.
Didelphys uterus sharing vagina.

Iron deficiency anaemia is a very prevalent condition in pregnancy, affecting nearly 18% of all pregnant women during all trimesters, with as many as 29% of women affected during the third trimester [25]. In twin pregnancies, the maternal iron demands are magnified, estimated at 1.8 times higher more than in singleton pregnancies [26], due to greater maternal red blood cell mass and plasma volume expansion as well as increased fetal and placental requirements. The maternal

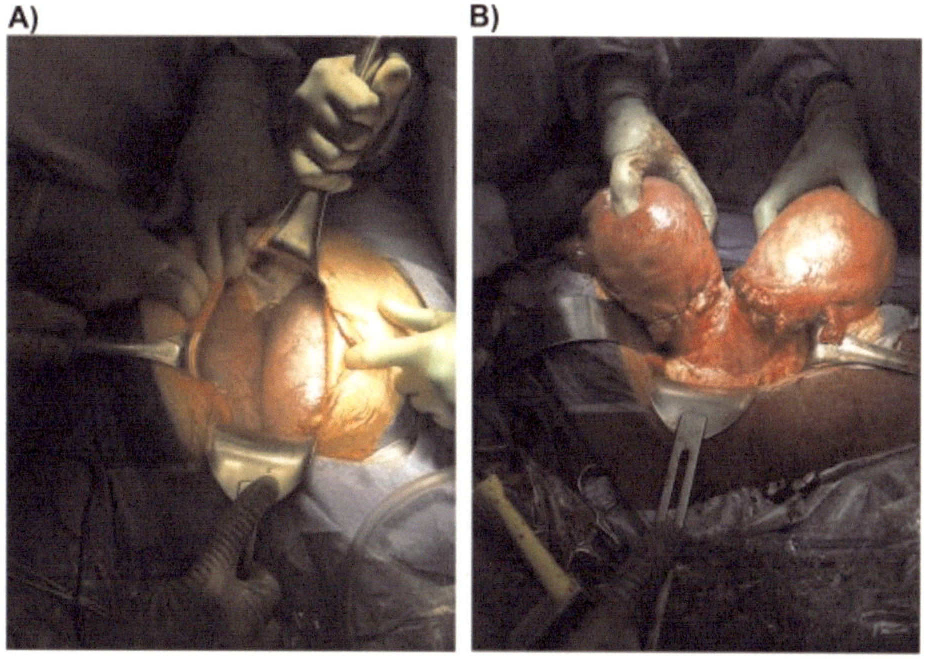

Figure 8.
Dicavitary twin pregnancy.

haemoglobin in multiple pregnancies is lower in all trimesters compared to singleton pregnancies.

Hypertensive disorders are among the most common complications occurring during pregnancy and one of the indication for admission with associated maternal and neonatal morbidity and mortality. The prevalence of preeclampsia is estimated to be 4.6% globally and in multiple pregnancies the prevalence is fourfold more than in singleton pregnancies. Multiple pregnancy is identified as a risk factor for preeclampsia. The predisposing factors implicated are larger placental mass and associated markedly elevated circulating placental markers [27]. Preeclampsia phenotypes appear to be different when comparing preeclampsia in singleton and multiple pregnancies as the documented known risks like advanced maternal age, Diabetes mellitus co-morbidity are not associated with preeclampsia in multiple pregnancies. Multiple pregnancy is therefore an independent risk factor for preeclampsia [28]. Screening for preeclampsia in multiple pregnancy is not effective as the markers used do not have references in these patients [29]. Preeclampsia is commonly associated with monochorionic placentation compared to dichorionic placentation [30].

The risk of developing gestational Diabetes mellitus during pregnancy might be variable according to the race, age, nutrition, pre-pregnancy rate or body mass index, familial history, hormonal and genetic factors. There are conflicting data regarding whether women with multiple pregnancy have higher risk of gestational Diabetes mellitus compared to women with singleton pregnancies. The expectation looking at the pathophysiology of gestational Diabetes mellitus based on the hormones of pregnancy that have insulin antagonist effects, gestational Diabetes in multiple pregnancy should be more common as these hormones are higher compared to singleton pregnancies. The other factors may be playing a role rather than multiple pregnancy alone [31].

3.3 Pregnancy specific complications

1. Preterm labour

2. Antepartum haemorrhage

3. Fetal weight

4. Fetal growth related

5. Polyhydramnios

6. Monochorionic specific

Antepartum haemorrhage occurs more frequently in twin pregnancy than in singleton pregnancies because of increased prevalence of preeclampsia in twin pregnancies with its associated placental abruption and the larger area of placental tissue with the likelihood of separation. There is no difference in the occurrence between monozygotic and dizygotic twins [31].

Twin-specific factors are zygosity, sex and birth order. Zygosity seems to play a role in intrauterine twin growth, with dizygotic twins being heavier than monozygotic twins [32]. Birth weight does not only depend on the sex of the twin but also on the sex of the co-twin. Gestation for females lasts longer than males, but despite their longer gestational age, birth weight of females is less than that for males [33].

Single intrauterine fetal demise in a twin pregnancy is a serious complication of pregnancy. It is a relatively rare complication of multiple pregnancy with a prevalence of 5–6% of all twin pregnancies [34, 35]. Single intrauterine demise during the first trimester is not an uncommon event and seems not to impair further development of the surviving one. This phenomenon is described as the "vanishing twin syndrome". The rate of disappearance in the first trimester could be as high as 29%. In contrast, the death of a twin in the late second trimester of pregnancy is a rare complication associated with increased maternal and fetal morbidity and mortality. This condition is highly associated with preterm labour, preeclampsia, intrauterine growth restriction of the surviving twin, neurological complications and even death as well as maternal disseminated intravascular coagulopathy [36]. Preterm delivery is the commonest adverse outcome occurring in more than 50% of twin pregnancies with a single fetal demise [35]. The dead twin may be reabsorbed by the body of the mother or be flattened against the side of the uterus by the sibling creating "fetus papyraceous" (**Figure 9**) [37].

Unique to multiple pregnancy gestation, discordance is the difference in the weights of the foetuses. Discordance is defined with the larger twin as the standard of growth and is calculated as: (larger estimated or actual weight –smaller estimated or actual weight)/larger estimated or actual weight. ACOG considers a 15–25% difference in actual weight among twins to be discordant. Risk factors for discordant growth are monochorionic twins, opposite sex of foetuses, and infrequent isolated transplacental viral infection [38].

Polyhydramnios refers to an excessive accumulation of amniotic fluid and is diagnosed when amniotic fluid index is more than 24 cm in the late second trimester or third trimester. Risk factors are fetal congenital anomalies, Diabetes mellitus, Rhesus isoimmunization, intrauterine infections and multiple pregnancy [39].

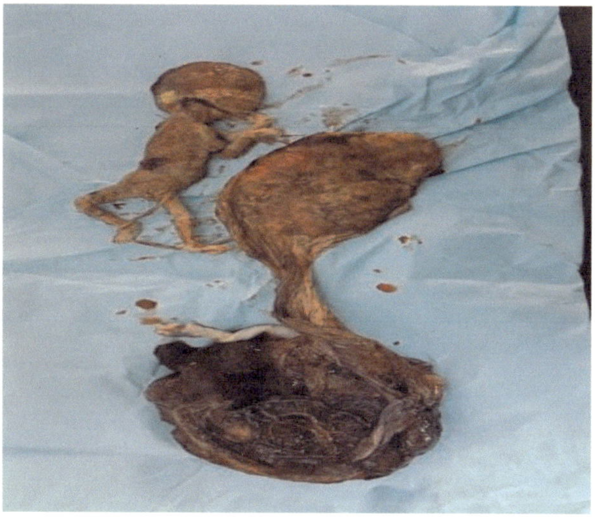

Figure 9.
Fetus papyraceus.

Polyhydramnios may be chronic or acute. Acute polyhydramnios is defined as a condition where the amniotic fluid exceeds 200mls or a standard deviation above the amount corresponding to the gestational age and as a rapid development of this increase within few days. This is often associated with monozygotic twin pregnancies. In monozygotic twin pregnancy, polyhydramnios is usually caused by unidirectional shunt between the two fetal circulations leading to anaemia of the donor and to polycythaemia of the recipient twin. The increased urine excretion of the hypervolaemic recipient twin results in "acute polyhydramnios" [40].

4. Monochorionc twins

Monochorionic diamniotic twins (**Figures 10–12**) presents with unique complications as a result of vascular malformations with shunts formation between the two foetuses.

4.1 Twin-twin transfusion syndrome

Twin-twin transfusion syndrome (TTTS) occurs in 10–15% of all monochorionic diamniotic twins. TTTS is a severe haemodynamic disorder characterised by hypovolaemia, oliguria of the donor twin and hypervolaemia, polyuria and polyhydramnios in the recipient. This is as a results of unbalanced bidirectional inter-twin blood flow. The severity depends on number and/or diameter of arteriovenous anastomoses from the donor to the recipient fetus.

4.2 Diagnostic criteria of TTTS is based on

1. Confirmed monochorionic pregnancy

2. polyhydramnios in the recipient with deepest vertical pool pocket ≥8 cm

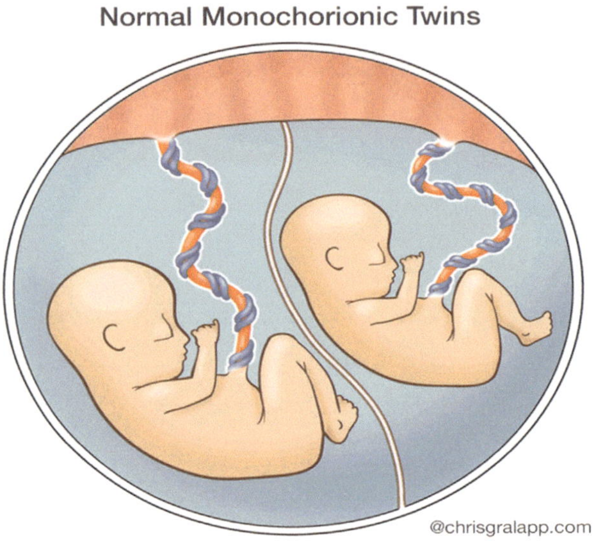

Figure 10.
Monochorinic twins.

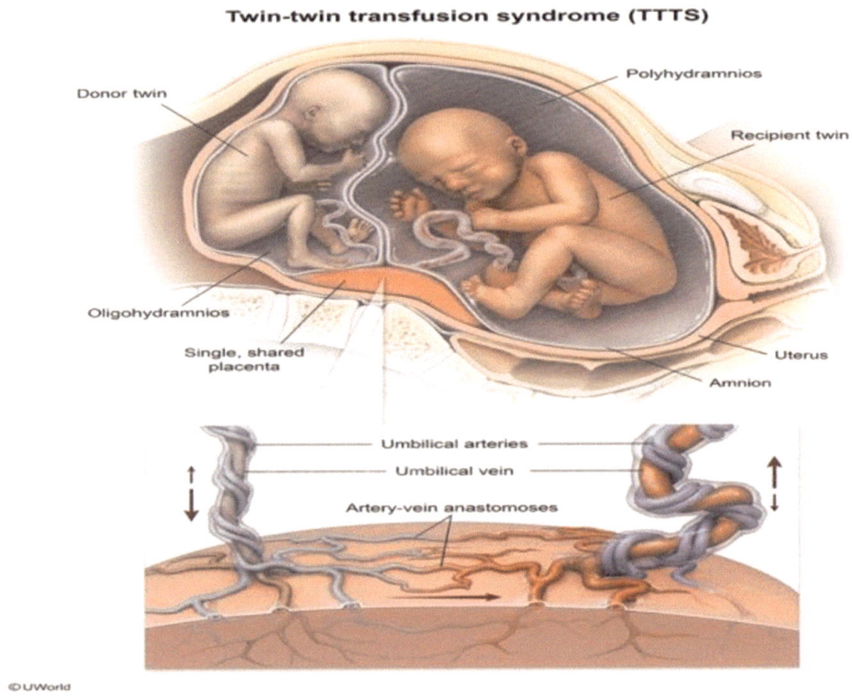

Figure 11.
Vascular anastomoses.

3. Oligohydramnios in the donor with a deepest vertical pool pocket ≤2 cm

4. Discordant fetal bladders with markedly enlarged bladder in the recipient and very small or non-visible in the donor.

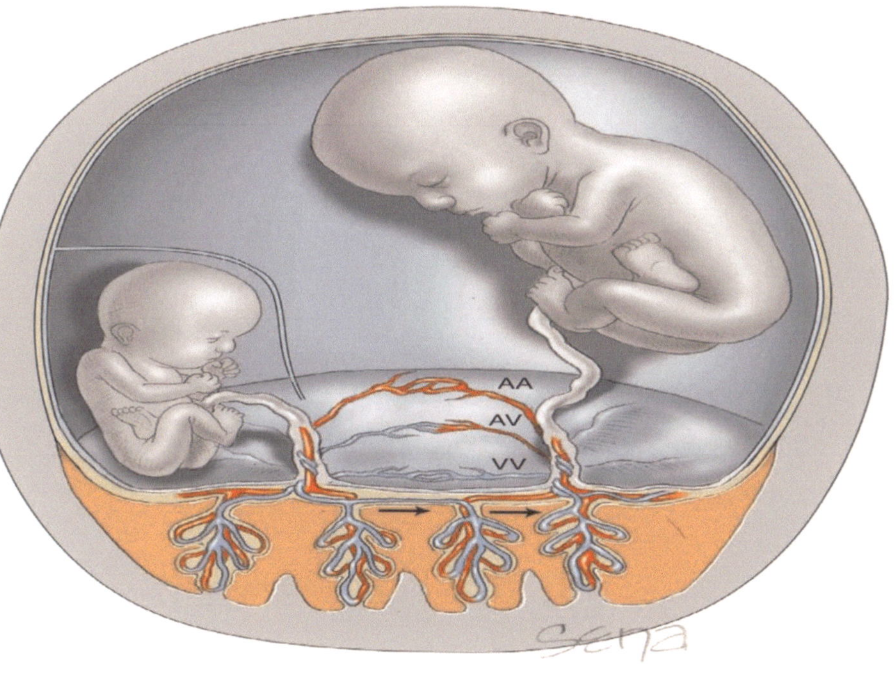

Figure 12.
Twin discordance.

4.3 Grading of severity of TTTS

Stage 1: The bladder is still visible in the donor
Stage 2: The bladder no visible in the donor
Stage 3: Critically abnormal Doppler in either twin: absent/reversed umbilical artery diastolic flow of the donor or recipient and/or absent/reversed ductus venosus flow or pulsatile flow in the umbilical vein of the recipient
Stage 4: Hydrops in either fetus
Stage 5: Demise in one or both foetuses.

4.4 Twin anaemic polycythaemis sequence

Twin anaemia polycythemia sequence (TAPS) (**Figure 13**) is a form of intertwine unbalanced transfusion occurring in a placenta where interfetal anastomoses are very small. It is a form of TTTS with reduced impact. Diagnostic criteria of TAPS is as in **Table 1** [41].

4.5 Twin reversed arterial (TRAP) perfusion

TRAP is defined as a degree of development of the fetus. It is classified according to specific organ with anomaly. The diagnosis has been made even in the first trimester in some cases using colour flow Doppler to document that the umbilical vein blood flow in the acardia twin goes from the twin to the placenta instead of the normal circulation which is from placenta to the fetus [42].

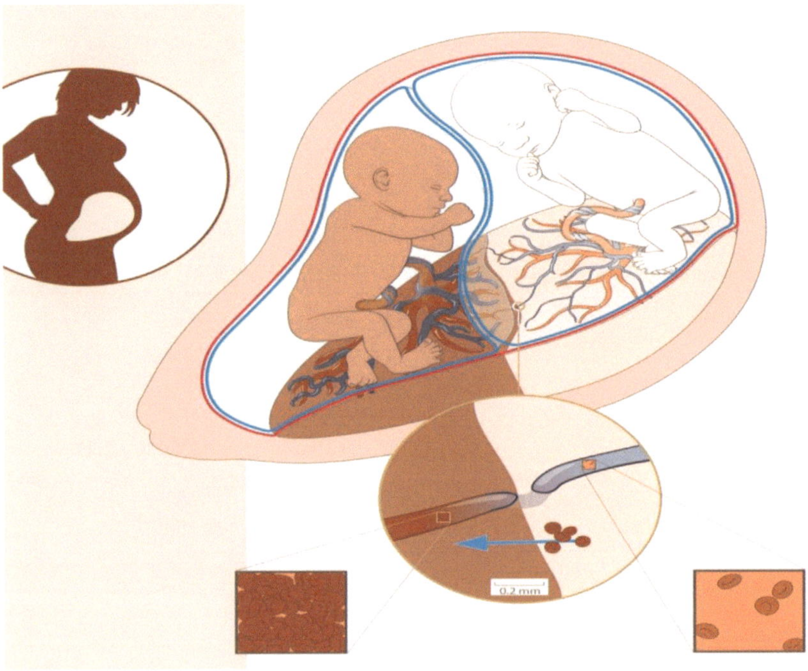

Figure 13.
Twin anaemic polycythaemic sequences (TAPS).

Malformed organ	Name
Failed head growth	Acardius acephalus
Malformed head and extremeties	Acardius myelacephalus
Rudimentary heart	hemicardius
Absent heart	Holocardius

Table 1.
Classification of TRAP.

4.6 Acute feto-fetal transfusion

This condition refers to sudden drop in pressure and/or heart rate at one fetal end. This leads to unidirectional transfusion and acute exsanguination of the co-twin which behaves like acute donation of blood. After a single fetal death, transfusion occurs from the surviving twin to the dead fetus. Acute feto-fetal transfusion by single intrauterine death is a rare condition in which blood transfusion from the surviving twin to the dying twin takes place. This may occur during pregnancy and delivery. If it occurs during pregnancy the surviving twin may suffer a massive exsanguination into the circulation of the dying twin. The surviving twin may suffer from brain injury and spontaneous death **Table 2** [41].

Prenatal	Middle cerebral artery (MCA) –peak systolic (PSV) ≥ 1.50 MoM in the anaemic fetus And MCA-PSV ≤ 0.8 MoM in the polycythaemic fetus Or Delta MCA-PSV ≥ 1.0 MoM
Postnatal	Inter-twin haemoglobin difference ≥ 8.0 g/dl And Inter-twin reticulocyte count ratio (anaemic/polycythaemic fetus) ≥ 1.7

Table 2.
Diagnostic criteria for TAPS.

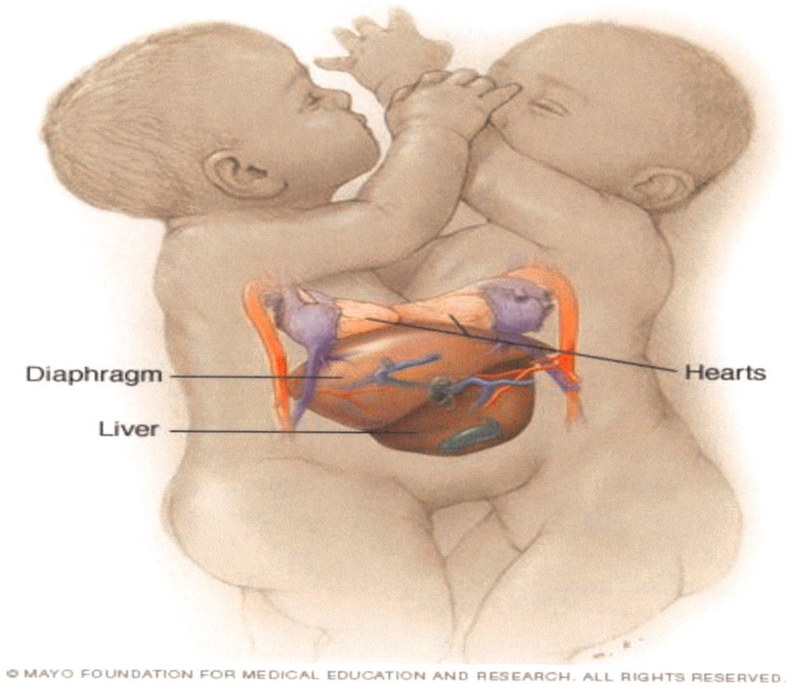

Figure 14.
Conjoined twins.

4.7 Conjoined twins

This is as a result of incomplete separation of monochorionic monoamniotic twins which should occur before eighth day after fertilisation. The points of union differ from the cephalic, thoracic, abdominal and caudal region. The incidence of conjoined twins is 1.5 per 100,000 deliveries and 50% of them are liveborns [43, 44]. The delivery is usually complicated as it should take place simultaneously and vaginal delivery is not possible (**Figure 14**).

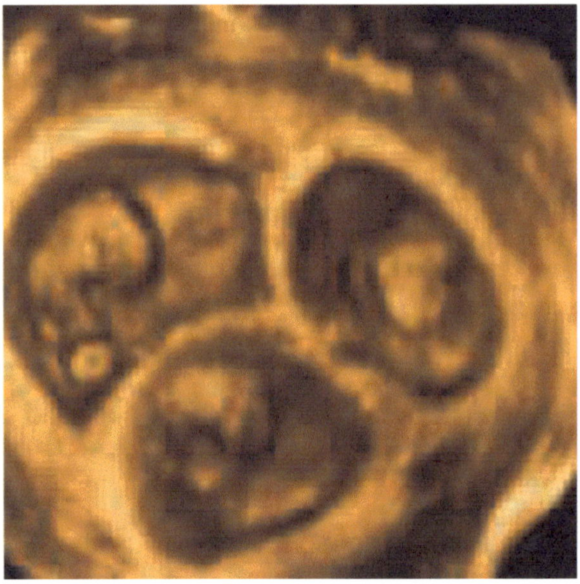

Figure 15.
Triplet pregnancy.

5. Higher order multiple pregnancy

This refers to a pregnancy with three or more foetuses. Though rare higher order multiple pregnancy have more serious complications than twin pregnancy. Preterm labour occurs at an earlier gestational age and lead to serious morbidity and increased maternal and neonatal mortality. Spontaneous miscarriages, preterm labour, preterm rupture of membranes, hypertensive disease in pregnancy, caesarean delivery, antepartum and postpartum haemorrhage are the anticipated challenges (**Figure 15**) [45].

6. Malpresentation

Malpresentation in multiple pregnancy is common as cephalic/cephalic presentation is estimated to be about 38–40% and vertex/non-vertex presentation accounts for approximately 34.8%. The general consensus is that a trial of vaginal delivery of vertex/vertex twins is appropriate at any gestational age. There is significant number of multiple pregnancies with abnormal presentation [46]. With abnormal presentation and abnormal fetal lie the option for delivery is surgical. The safest delivery mode of twins has been controversial as there has reported that postpartum haemorrahage is more often after vaginal delivery than after elective caesarean section. Elective caesarean section delivery is relatively safe for twin pregnancy, because the second twin in vaginal delivery has a high probability of birth injuries and death [45].

7. Postpartum haemorrhage

Uterine over-distension as in multiple pregnancy and singleton with large foetuses more than 4000 g is associated with uterine atony. In addition, the large placental size in multiple pregnancy increases the surface area for bleeding after delivery [47]. Multiple pregnancy and caesarean section are well known risks factors for postpartum haemorrhage. Comorbidity in multiple pregnancy like hypertensive disorders increase the risk of postpartum haemorrhage even higher.

Growth discordance, especially complicated by fetal growth restriction is associated with increased risk of postpartum haemorrhage in women with twin pregnancies undergoing caesarean section, and more so in patients with dichorionic twins [48].

Low platelet counts of less than 100,000/ul was also identified as one of the risk factors for postpartum haemorrhage in twin pregnancy who had elective procedure even without hypertension. Preoperative measurement of platelet counts is clinically useful for predicting the occurrence of postpartum haemorrhage in caesarean section for twins. Optimization of platelet counts may reduce the risk [49].

8. Maternal and neonatal mortality

The occurrence of severe maternal morbidity and maternal death is significantly higher among twin compared to singleton pregnancies [50]. Twin delivery has a negative impact on perinatal health indicators, since the mortality is higher, especially due to higher preterm births. Early neonatal mortality may be as high as seven times higher among twins compared to singletons. Morbidity and mortality of the second twin and subsequent foetuses in higher multiple pregnancy is even higher than the first, particularly for non-cephalic presentation [51, 52].

9. Conclusion

Multiple pregnancy poses challenges from conception until delivery. The delay of women in reproduction leads to the need of assisted reproductive techniques to be implemented increasing the prevalence of multiple pregnancy including higher order. The impact of multiple pregnancy on maternal and neonatal morbidity and increased cost to manage is enormous. Complications of multiple pregnancy are noticed early in pregnancy and continue to be present throughout pregnancy and delivery until in the postpartum period. Multiple pregnancy is significantly associated with severe maternal morbidity associated with worse perinatal outcome. Neonatal morbidity and mortality are significant in multiple pregnancy presenting challenges for health services.

Acknowledgements

The completion of this undertaking could not have been possible without the help of my daughter Unarine Mashamba. Her contribution is sincerely appreciated and gratefully acknowledged.

Author details

Tshililo Mashamba
Department of Obstetrics and Gynaecology, Sefako Makgatho University, Pretoria, South Africa

*Address all correspondence to: tjmashamba@yahoo.com

References

[1] Katke RD, Thakre NN. Multifetal pregnancy: Maternal and neonatal outcome. Obstetrics and Gynecology International. 2015;**3**(1):229-234

[2] Kazandi M, Turan V. Multiple pregnancies and their complications (review). Journal of Turkish Society of Obstetric and Gynecology. 2011;**8**(1): 21-14

[3] Balassiano K, Malik S, Vaid P, et al. The presence of multiple gestational sacs confers a higher live birth rate in women with infertility who achieve a positive pregnancy test after fresh and frozen embryo transfer; a retrospective local cohort. Reproductive Biology and Endocrinology. 2014;**12**:104

[4] Livingston JE, Poland BJ. A study of spontaneously aborted twins. Teratology. 1980;**21**:139-148

[5] Urchida IA, Freman VC, Gedeon M, Goldmaker J. Twin rate in spontaneous abortions. American Journal of Human Genetics. 1983;**35**(5):987-993

[6] Ji W, Hou B, Li W, Guo F, He P, Zheng J. Associations between first trimester intrauterine hematoma and twin pregnancy outcomes: A retrospective cohort study. BMC Pregnancy and Childbirth. 2021;**21**:46

[7] Keoldrup L, Larsen LA, Fagerberg C, Hertz JM, Christensen K. Chromosomal aberrations in monozygotic and dizygotic twins versus singletons in Denmark during 1968-2009. Twin Research and Human Genetics. 2017; **20**(3):216-225

[8] Boyle B, Morris JK, Garne E, Loane M, Addor MC, Gatt M, et al. Prevalence and risk of down syndrome in monozygotic and dizygotic multiple pregnancies in Europe: Implications for prenatal screening. BJOG. 2014;**121**: 809-820

[9] Sperling L, Kiil C, Larsen LU, Brocks V, Wojdemanns QI, Schwartz M, et al. Detection of chromosomal abnormalities, congenital abnormalities and transfusion syndrome in twins. Ultrasound in Obstetrics & Gynecology. 2007;**29**:517-526

[10] Glinianaia SV, Rankin J, Wright C. Congenital anomalies in twins: A register-based study. Human Reproduction. 2008;**23**(6):1306-1311

[11] Jones KL. Smith's Recognizable Patterns of Human Malformation. Philadelphia, PA: Elsevier; 2006

[12] Ali T, Tawab MA, ELHariri MAG, Ayad AA. Heterotopic pregnancy: A case report. Egyptian Journal of Radiology and Nuclear Medicine. 2020;**51**:214

[13] Nabi U, Yousaf A, Ghaffar F, Sajid S, Ahmed MMH. Heterotopic pregnancy-a diagnostic challenge. Six case reports and literature review. Cureus. 2019;**11**(11):1-8

[14] Basile F, Di Cesare C, Quagliozzi L, Donati L, Bracaglia M, Caruso A, et al. Spontaneous heterotopic pregnancy, simultaneous ovarian and intrauterine: A case report. Case Reports in Obstetrics and Gynecology. 2012;**2012**:1-4

[15] Ghike S, Somalwar S, Mitra K, Kulkarni S, Ladikar M, Baisakhiya N, et al. Unilateral twin ectopic pregnancy (diamniotic-Dichorionic): A rare case. Journal of South Asian Federation of Obstetrics and Gynaecology. 2011;**3**(2): 103-105

[16] Madaan S, Jaiswal A, Banode P, Dhok A, Dewani D. Spontaneous twin

ectopic pregnancy managed successfully with methotrexate-mediated ultrasound-guided fetal reduction: A fertility preserving approach. Cureus. 2021;**13**(8):1-4

[17] Goswami D, Agrawal N, Arora V. Twin tubal pregnancy: A large unruptured ectopic pregnancy. Journal of Obstetrics and Gynaecology Research. 2015;**41**(11):1820-1822

[18] Badegheish A, Vilos AG, Baglaf H, Rafeh JA, Alzawawi N, Abu-Rafea B, et al. Reproductive and neonatal outcomes in women with unicornuate uterus: A population study. Obstetrics & Gynecology International Journal. 2021;**12**(5):344-350

[19] Al Yaqoubi HN, Fatema N. Successful vaginal delivery of naturally conceived dicavitary twin in didelphys uterus: A rare reported case. Hindawi. Case Reports in Obstetrics and Gynecology. 2017;**2017**:1-4

[20] Hafizi L, Ghomian N. Twin pregnancy in the unicornuate uterus and non-communicating rudimentary horn: A case report. International Journal of Reproductive BioMedicine. 2019;**17**(1):67-70

[21] Okonta PI, Abedi H, Ajuyah C, Omo-Aghoja. Pregnancy in a noncommunicating rudimentary horn of a unicornuate uterus: A case report. Cases Journal. 2009;**3**(6624):1-3

[22] King AL, Pixton S, Lanzarone V. Uterine didelphys with dicavitary twin gestation: A case report. Case Reports in Women's Health. 2020;**27**:1-3

[23] Levy G, Mottet N, Fourel M, Tholozan A, Eckman A, Ramanah R, et al. Twin pregnancy in each half of a didelphys uterus with delayed delivery and review of literature. Science Open Research. 2015:115-117

[24] Ozyyuncu O, Turgal M, Yazicioglu A, Ozek A. Spontaneous twin gestation in each horn of uterus didelphys complicated with unilateral preterm labour. Case Reports in Perinatal Medicine. 2014;**3**(1):53-56

[25] Bailit JL, Doty E, Todia W. Repeated hematocrit measurements in low-risk pregnant women. Journal of Reproductive Medicine. 2007;**52**:619-622

[26] Shinar S, Skornick-Rapaport A, Maslovitz S. Iron supplementation in twin pregnancy-the benefit of doubling the iron dose in iron deficient pregnant women: A randomized control trial. Twin Research and Human Genetics. 2017;**20**(5):419-424

[27] Laine K, Murzakanova G, Sole KB, Pay AD, Heradstveit S, Raisanen S. Prevalence and risk of pre-eclampsia and gestational hypertension in twin pregnancies: A population –based register study. BMJ Open. 2019;**9**:1-8

[28] Bergman L, Nordof-Callbo P, Wikstrom K, Snowden JM, Hesslman S, Bonamy EKE, et al. Multi-Fetal pregnancy, preeclampsia, and long-term cardiovascular disease. Hypertension. 2020;**76**(1):1-12

[29] Chen J, Zhao D, Liu Y, Zhou J, Zou G, Zhang Y, et al. Screening for preclampsia in low-risk twin pregnancies at early gestation. Acta Obstetricia et Gynecologica Scandinavica. 2020;**99**:1346-1353

[30] Campbell D. Twin Research. 2001;**4**(3):146-149

[31] Kim Y, Hong S, Kim Y, Sung J, Choi S, Oh S, et al. Obstetric and neonatal outcomes of gestational

diabetes mellitus in twin pregnancies according to changes in its diagnostic criteria from National Diabetes Data Group criteria to carpenter and Coustan criteria: A retrospective cohort study. BMC Pregnancy and Childbirth. 2022;**22**:9

[32] Christensen K, Vaupel JW, Holm NV, Yashin AI. Mortality among twins after age 6: Fetal origins hypothesis versus twin method. BMJ. 1995;**310**: 432-436

[33] Morley R, Dwyer T. Studies of twins: What can they tell us about the fetal origins of adult disease? Paediatric and Perinatal Epidemiology. 2005;**19**(Suppl 1):2-7

[34] Reddy AC, Vasanthalakshmi GN. Single intrauterine fetal demise in twin pregnancies and pregnancy outcomes. The Journal of South Asian Federation of Obstetrics and Gynaecology. 2021;**13**(3): 137-141

[35] Mackie FL, Rigby A, Kilby MD. Prognosis of the co-twin following spontaneous single intrauterine fetal death in twin pregnancies: A systematic review and meta-analysis. BJOG. 2019; **126**:569-578

[36] Stefanescu BI, Adam A-M, Constantin GB, Trus C. Single fetal demise in twin pregnancy-a great concern but still a favorable outcome. Diseases. 2021;**9**(33):1-9

[37] Tayade S, Kumar N. Demise of co-twin in second trimester leading to fetus papyraceous-successful outcome in surviving twin. IJBR. 2012;**3**(5):268-270

[38] American College of Obstetricians and Gynecologists' Committee on Practice Bulletins—Obstetrics, Society for Maternal-Fetal Medicine. Multifetal Gestations: Twin, Triplet, and Higher-Order Multifetal Pregnancies: ACOG Practice Bulletin, Number 231. Obstetrics and Gynecology, 2021;**137**(6): 1118-1132

[39] Tshfeen K, Hamdi IM. Polyhydramnios as a predictor of adverse pregnancy outcomes. SQUMJ. 2013;**13**(1):57-62

[40] Schneider KTM, Vetter K, Huch A. Acute polyhydramnios complicating twin pregnancies. Acta Geneticae Medicae et Gemellologiae. 1985;**34**: 179-184

[41] Mitchletti T, Eixarch E, Bennasar M, Martinez JM, Gratacos E. Complications of monochorionic diamniotic twins: Stepwise approach for early identification, differential diagnosis, and clinical management. Maternal-Fetal Medicine. 2020;**3**(1):42-52

[42] Langlotz H, Sauerbrei E, Murray S. Transvaginal Doppler sonographic diagnosis of an acardiac twin at 12 weeks gestation. Journal of Ultrasound in Medicine. 1991;**10**:175-179

[43] Chambliss LR. Twin reversed arterial perfusion in one foetus in a triplet pregnancy with a singleton foetus and dichorionic monoamniotic twins conceived with in vitro fertilization: A case report. Obstetrics and Gynecology Reports. 2020;**4**:1-4

[44] Liu H, Deng C, Hu Q, Liao H, Wang X, Yu H. Conjoined twins in dichorionic diamniotic triplet pregnancy: A report of three cases and literature review. BMC Pregnancy and Childbirth. 2021;**21**(687):s12884-s12021

[45] Oriji VK, Nyeche SN. Adverse maternal outcomes in high-order multiple pregnancies in a private health facility in Nigeria: A 10-year experience. JBM. 2020;**8**:103-110

[46] Cruikshank DP. Intrapartum management of twin gestation. Obstetrics & Gynecology. 2007;**109**: 1167-1176

[47] Yang Q, Wen SW. Neonatal mortality and morbidity in vertex-vertex second twins according to mode of delivery and birth weight. Journal of Perinatology. 2006;**26**:3-10

[48] Ononge S, Mirembe F, Wandabwa J, et al. Incidence and risk factors for postpartum hemorrhage in Uganda. Reproductive Health. 2016;**13**(38):1-7

[49] Cao X, Luo Y, Zhou S, Zhao Q, Qin X, Liu Z, et al. Frontiers in Medicine. 2022;**9**:1-8

[50] Shibata Y, Miyazaki M, Hayashi Z, Suzuki S. Influence of platelet counts on postpartum hemorrhage in elective cesarean section for Japanese twins. Hypertens Res Pregnancy. 2021;**9**:51-54

[51] Danielly S, Silveira C, Costa ML, Souza RT, Surita FG, Souza JP, et al. Perinatal outcomes in twin pregnancies complicated by maternal morbidity: Evidence from the WHO multicountry survey on maternal and Newborn health. BMC Pregnancy and Childbirth. 2018; **18**(449):2082-2089

[52] Esteves-Pereira AP, da Cunha, Nakamura-Pereira M, Moreira ME, RMSM D, Viellas EF. Twin pregnancy and perinatal outcomes. PLoS One. 2021; **16**(1):1-13